I0456595

SHATTER & SCATTER THE LIES

ACQUIRING TRUTH: GIVING A VOICE TO CHILDHOOD TRAUMA

JOANNE GAIL RICHARDSON

Copyright © 2025 by Joanne Gail Richardson

Paperback ISBN: 979-8-9941249-0-1

All Worldwide Rights Reserved.
All rights reserved. No part of this book may be reproduced, stored in a retrieval system or
transmitted, in any form or by any means, electronic, mechanical, recorded, photocopied, or
otherwise, without the prior written permission of the copyright owner, except by a reviewer
who may quote brief passages in a review.

CONTENTS

FORWARD

Joanne Richardson's self-help workbook, *Acquiring Truth: Shattering and Scattering the Lies*, is a deeply personal account of one woman's reflections on endurance, redemption, atonement, faith, and salvation. It is beautifully written with heartfelt wisdom and empathy; her prose is poetry.

The workbook was written from the point of view of a heroic survivor of Complex Post-Traumatic Stress Disorder (CPTSD). It is an excellent self-guided workbook that focuses on empowerment, the process of gaining freedom to take authority over yourself and empower you to make decisions for yourself that align with your goals, not someone else's goal for you.

If you have abdicated your self-worth, been manipulated by someone else to feel hopeless, helpless, and powerless, help is on the way. If you are tangled in endless, unwarranted phantom shame and guilt, this workbook is for you. If you have lied to yourself and morphed into a stranger to please others and seek their love, look for your truth in the pages of this workbook.

Acquiring Truth: Shattering and Scattering the Lies is suitable for anyone looking for guidance and new perspectives on old problems. It is a safe, self-paced start for those who are hesitant to start psychotherapy. Therapists will find it a welcome addition to their Therapist's Toolbox.

Dr. Carolyn Greenleaf, LCSW

Christian Therapist I Trauma and Resilience Specialist

BEFORE YOU BEGIN

I wrote this workbook for anyone who's tired of pretending they're fine. You don't have to know my story to use this—you just need the courage to face yours. I've spent years unpacking trauma, betrayal, silence, and survival. What I learned is this: healing doesn't happen by accident. It happens when you stop running from yourself. This isn't a workbook full of fluffy affirmations or quick fixes. It's a mirror, a reckoning, and an invitation to tell the truth—to yourself first. If you've ever felt like you were too much, not enough, or always stuck playing a part just to be accepted, this is your space to call it out and change it. Not for them. For you.

You can't afford to keep carrying what was never yours to begin with. The pain you've buried hasn't disappeared—it's just been leaking into your relationships, your decisions, your silence, your self-worth. This workbook is about cleaning the wound, not covering it. You may not want to look back. You may think you've moved on. But if your past still controls your present, you haven't healed—you've adapted. That's not freedom. That's survival. And you deserve more than that. This work is hard. It will pull things out of you. But if you finish it, you won't be the same person who started.

If you show up for this process fully—no filters, no pretending—you will not leave the same. You will see things clearly: where the pain began, what it cost you, and what you've been dragging behind you without realizing it. You'll start to separate who you are from what happened to you. The shame that felt permanent will start to lose its grip. The habits, the roles, the silence—they'll start to make sense. And once you name something, you can stop being ruled by it. This isn't a fix. It's a fracture followed by reset. But it's real. And you'll feel it. You'll know it when the weight shifts, when your voice returns, when you stop apologizing for existing. That's healing—and it's possible. If you're ready, it's yours.

A Note on Safety & Pacing

This workbook is raw on purpose. It names silence, shame, betrayal, abuse, and grief. Some chapters will stir memories you've buried or feelings you've been taught to minimize. That doesn't mean you're weak—it means you're human. Healing starts with telling the truth.

But telling the truth also stirs pain. So before you dive in, here's how to protect yourself as you work through these pages:

1. Go slow. This is not a sprint. One or two chapters a week is enough. Let the prompts breathe. If you feel pressure to "finish," pause—that's survival mode talking.

2. Check your state. Think in traffic lights:

> **Green:** calm, steady—you're ready to reflect.
> **Yellow:** edgy, restless—slow down, ground yourself.
> **Red:** overwhelmed, spiraling—close the book, breathe, return later.

There is no prize for pushing through red.

3. Use grounding tools. When emotions spike, try this:

• Look around and name 5 things you see, 4 you can touch, 3 you hear, 2 you smell, 1 you taste.

• Put your hand on your heart and breathe in for 4, hold 4, out for 6.

• Pray a short truth: *"I am safe. God is with me. I can stop now."*

4. Notice triggers.

Some chapters (suicidality, abuse, estrangement) may be heavy. Read the content advisories and decide if you're in a safe enough place before continuing. Skipping a section is not failure—it's wisdom.

5. Bring community.

This workbook can be done alone, but healing deepens with safe people. Share what you're ready to share with a trusted friend, therapist, pastor, or group. You don't owe anyone every detail.

6. Crisis plan.

If your pain ever feels unbearable, please reach out:

- **U.S.: dial or text 988** (Suicide & Crisis Lifeline)
- Call your doctor, therapist, or a trusted friend immediately
- If you are in immediate danger, call 911 (U.S.) or your local emergency number

You are not alone. Your presence matters—even on the days you can't feel it. You didn't cause your trauma. But you do get to choose your healing.

Go slow. Tell the truth. Rest when you need to. Come back when you're ready.

This is not about perfection. It's about peace.

PREFACE

TO THE ONE WHO IS READY TO HEAL

Who I Am — And Who I Am Not

I am not a psychologist, therapist, or mental-health professional. I hold no degrees in psychiatry or clinical counseling. I do not diagnose, prescribe, or speak from academic theory.

What I am is a woman with lived Complex PTSD — decades of it — carved into my body, my reactions, my relationships, and my faith. I come to this work not from textbooks, but from the trenches of trauma and the slow rebuilding that only God could guide me through. Everything I share in these pages was learned through lived experience, through prayer, through breaking, and through being rebuilt by Christ one surrendered moment at a time.

I know what it feels like to have a story you can barely hold. I know the exhaustion of being triggered by things you don't understand. I know the confusion of wondering why you react so intensely... and the shame of thinking something is "wrong" with you when really, something happened to you.

This workbook was created for people who carry wounds that never healed the first time. People who have learned to survive instead of feel.

People who want to heal but don't know where to begin. And I want you to hear this clearly: *you are not broken — you are affected.*

CPTSD is the body and brain's long-term response to repeated trauma, abandonment, neglect, emotional injury, or environments that taught you to suppress your truth in order to stay safe. It can feel like hyper-vigilance, emotional overwhelm, numbness, shame, people-pleasing, anger, self-doubt, or the internal belief that you're "too much." It can feel like living in a body that remembers what your mind tried to forget.

This workbook does not replace therapy — it sits beside it. It is a companion for the heart, a guide for reflection, and a place to breathe when everything in you wants to shut down. It is crafted with empathy, with honesty, and with the understanding that every step toward healing is sacred.

I am a survivor, a seeker of truth, and a woman who was carried through the fire by the Holy Spirit. And as you move through these pages, I want you to feel seen, understood, and honored — not judged.

I walk with you not as an expert looking down, but as someone who has lived this, healed through Christ, and believes with my whole heart that God can restore what trauma tried to destroy.

You are safe here.

Take your time.

You're not alone anymore.

PART I

Survival Patterns

Before you could heal, you had to survive. Survival doesn't ask if it's healthy — it just asks if it works. You learned to go silent, to overachieve, to disappear, to please, to fight, to control, to disguise. Some of those patterns kept you alive, but they also cost you pieces of yourself. This Stage pulls those patterns into the light. Not to shame you, but to help you see them for what they are: survival, not identity.

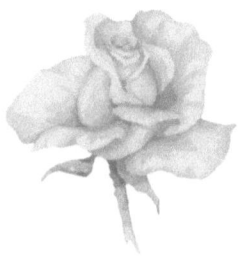

THE MIRROR DOESN'T LIE—BUT IT DOESN'T HEAL EITHER

CONFRONTING SELF-IMAGE, IDENTITY, AND THE ROOTS OF SHAME

*I*t all begins with something we all do: we check the mirror.

We fix what's visible, assess the damage, and pull ourselves together before stepping out. But here's the truth: the mirror can only show what's on the surface. It won't tell you why you look tired. It won't explain the fear in your eyes or the tension in your jaw. It won't reveal the years you've spent holding your breath just to survive.

It reflects, but it doesn't restore.

Some of us have used the mirror as a weapon, others as a disguise. We tried to control the reflection because we couldn't control the pain underneath it. But at some point, you have to stop asking your reflection for answers it was never built to give.

This section isn't about how you look. It's about who you are when no one's watching. It's about the layers beneath what you've learned to project, and whether you're finally ready to face the parts of you that don't fit into a filter. Let's start there—not with the mirror, but with you.

We begin at childhood, because that's where your story began—whether you remember it clearly or not. Our earliest years shape the way we see ourselves, others, and the world. Before we had language for pain, we had reactions. Before we understood manipulation, we learned to perform. The roles we play, the shame we carry, the triggers we can't explain—all of it traces back to those first imprints.

You might think you've outgrown the past, but unresolved wounds don't stay buried. They drive behavior, distort relationships, and sabotage healing. This isn't about blaming your upbringing. It's about tracing the roots so you can stop watering the weeds. Childhood wasn't just a beginning. For many, it was the blueprint for survival—and it's time to rewrite it.

~

What were you called as a child—and what did you start calling yourself because of it?

Not nicknames. Labels—the ones that stuck, the ones that still whisper. Who told you who you were? Who assigned names to your identity? Who tore you down? Who built you up?

_____

_____

_____

What part of yourself did you hide to stay safe, loved, or accepted?

Trace it back. Who made you feel like you were "too much"? When did you learn to edit yourself? Who did you fear? Who made your voice small? Who treated you like a precious gift?

_____

_____

_____

What role did you play in your family or early life that you've never stopped performing?

Caretaker, achiever, peacemaker, rebel—write the script you've been reciting. Was it ever really you? Are you in a role within your family you didn't ask for? How would it feel to step out from under your family's perception of you—or even your own?

_____

_____

_____

What's the earliest moment you remember feeling ashamed of who you were—not what you did, but who you were?

Where were you? What did you believe about yourself in that moment? Did you feel humiliation or rage? Do those words or actions still cling to you today? Something you can't seem to forget?

_____

_____

_____

What image of yourself have you carried for so long, it feels like truth—but it's not?

Is it strong-but-alone? Smart-but-unlovable? Quiet-but-boiling? Who gave you that image? Maybe it was you. Maybe you decided it was easier to step into a mask than face the truth of your circumstances.

_____

_____

_____

What do you still believe about yourself that someone broken taught you?

This isn't blame. It's exposure. Name what they projected—and what you've carried.

_____

_____

_____

If your younger self could see your life now, what would they recognize—and what would break their heart?

Write it as a letter. Let the child in you speak.

_____

_____

_____

Now Step Back and Look

Take a breath. Read your own words—especially the names—out loud if you can. This is where things start to shift: when you stop seeing your identity as something that happened to you and start owning the part you play in keeping it alive.

Maybe you became the peacemaker to avoid conflict, or the perfectionist so no one would criticize you. Maybe you learned to disappear. Maybe you learned to dominate. Maybe you became the one who needed control, or the one who always gave it away. Are you still playing small to make others comfortable? Still letting pain write your story? Still wearing labels someone else stuck to your skin?

Maybe you've become the fixer, the addict, the one who absorbs everyone else's damage just so you don't have to feel your own. Whatever version of yourself you see on these pages, don't look away. You're not being shamed—you're being seen.

This is your turning point. But nothing turns if you don't face it first.

When I first started putting my outline together for this book, I began at my mirror—not as a metaphor, but the actual mirror I stood in front of, covered in the tiles I placed. Each one held a story. A lie I believed. A name I was given. A role I performed. I had created quite an elaborate showcase—layer after layer—to reflect the image I thought the world wanted from me.

But none of it showed the real me.

When I finally looked closer, I saw it. The mirror didn't reflect my soul. It reflected survival. So I started pulling the tiles back—one by one. Behind them was self-doubt, self-betrayal, the truth of how far I'd fallen. Not professionally. Not socially. But emotionally. Spiritually. Internally.

The stories I had buried to keep my image intact were horrifying to look at. But I had to see them, because those tiles weren't just decoration—they were evidence. Evidence of how I'd been taught to see myself. Evidence of what I'd hidden. Evidence of what had to be unlearned if I was ever going to write this book in truth.

My mirror—my real one—became the starting point. The mirror of self-reflection, of soul state, of honesty. And what I saw staring back wasn't just painful. It was the truth. That mirror and those tiles became the backbone of this entire book. Every chapter, every prompt, every story starts there.

This wasn't about writing a book. This was about pulling off the lies and finally seeing what was underneath.

Right Decisions Honesty Respect Benevolence LOYALTY HONOR VALOR | 7 Bushido Virtues

Abstinence Kindness Humility Liberality CHASTITY Patience Diligence | 7 Contrary Virtues

FAITH CHARITY FORTITUDE PRUDENCE Temperance HOPE Justice | 7 Heavenly Virtues

Gluttony ENVY PRIDE GREED LUST WRATH SLOTH | 7 DEADLY

FOOD Alcohol Shopping IMAGE WORK | SEX | SELF HATRED Depression | ISMs

Drugs

Ill HEALTH EMPTY Desperation Worry | USED UP Suicide BROKEN | SATAN

2

WHEN SILENCE BECOMES SURVIVAL

EXPLORING FAMILY DYNAMICS, EMOTIONAL SUPPRESSION, AND SPEAKING YOUR TRUTH

*S*peaking your truth begins with this: silence isn't always peace. Sometimes it's protection. Sometimes it's punishment. And sometimes it was the only option you had.

If you grew up in a home where emotions weren't safe, you already know how silence becomes survival. You learned to bite your tongue, to read the room before you spoke, to bury the truth before anyone noticed it. Maybe you watched people explode when honesty got too close. Maybe you became the one who soothed everyone else just to avoid the fallout.

But here's what they didn't tell you: the silence you used to survive will strangle you if you keep living by it. You can't speak your truth while still obeying the rules that taught you to hide it. And you can't heal while still protecting the people who hurt you.

This section is about the emotional contracts you signed without even realizing it—the ones that said, "Don't upset them," "Keep the secret," "Be the strong one," and "Stay quiet and you'll stay safe." Maybe those agreements kept you alive once, but they're not keeping you free.

What were you taught—directly or indirectly—about expressing emotions in your family?

Were certain feelings allowed? Were others punished? Who was allowed to be angry? Who had to stay calm? Who exploded? Who disappeared?

_____

_____

_____

What did you witness growing up that made you believe silence was safer than truth?

Was it yelling? Was it withdrawal? Was it rejection? Were emotions turned into weapons—or ignored altogether?

_____

_____

_____

When was the first time you swallowed the truth to keep the peace?

Who did you protect? What did it cost you? What did you learn about your voice in that moment?

_____

_____

_____

Have you ever told a version of your story that left the hardest parts out?

Who were you trying to protect—yourself or someone else? What would it feel like to tell the whole truth?

_____

_____

_____

What do you still avoid saying because you know it will cause conflict or disappointment?

Write it down here. Say it in a sentence. Say it for you.

_____

_____

_____

Who taught you that honesty equals betrayal?

Who benefits when you stay silent? Who would lose power if you finally spoke?

_____

_____

_____

What has your silence protected—and what has it destroyed?

Be honest. Think of the cost. Think of what your silence has kept alive —and what it's killed.

_____

_____

_____

Now Step Back and Look

Silence has a cost, and now you're starting to see it. You didn't speak because you didn't want to hurt anyone, but somewhere along the way you learned that meant hurting yourself instead. You told yourself it wasn't the right time, that they wouldn't understand, that maybe it wasn't that bad, that maybe it was your fault.

That's what trauma does: it teaches you to minimize your own truth so others don't have to confront theirs. But you can't keep carrying that lie and expect to heal. You were never meant to hold their secrets. You were never meant to absorb their dysfunction. You were never meant to be the one who kept it all together by falling apart silently.

If something you wrote on these pages made your heart pound, that's your signal—the truth rising up. Let it come. Your voice was never the problem. Their comfort was never worth your silence. Your healing will never come from protecting someone else's image. This is your moment to choose truth over peacekeeping. You've done enough surviving. Now it's time to speak.

I had been conditioned early on to be silent, to be invisible, to not ask for too much, not be too needy, and to always give—even when it wasn't asked for and even when it drained me dry. Approval was never guaranteed; it was earned. I found myself running a race for acceptance I didn't remember signing up for—but somehow never stopped running.

I was taught that quiet meant strength, that silence was safe, that love was conditional and transactional, and that the currency was self-sacrifice. I learned to hold it all in because hurting myself felt safer than risking the chance of hurting someone else. And that self-harm—holding myself small and silent—was rewarded, applauded, expected. I just wanted to be a good girl.

Writing this chapter forced me to face what that silence cost me. It made me revisit every time I swallowed the truth to protect someone who never protected me. It asked me to admit how much I still minimize, still freeze, still fall into the trap of disappearing in order to be liked.

This wasn't just reflection. It was a reckoning. It started with pulling off the tile that said, "Don't speak. You'll ruin everything."

3

BURNING BRIDGES—OR BUILDING BOUNDARIES

UNDERSTANDING PERSONAL LIMITS

*R*edefining what it means to walk away—for good reason—starts with this truth: there's a difference between burning a bridge out of rage and walking away because you've finally had enough. But not everyone will see it that way. Especially not the people who benefited from your silence, your flexibility, and your constant return.

They'll call it dramatic. They'll call it unforgiving. They'll call it betrayal. But here's what they won't call it: overdue. Because boundaries don't just protect your peace—they expose who was violating it all along. Once you stop bending, people who relied on your flexibility will call you rigid. Once you stop over-giving, they'll call you selfish. Once you walk away, they'll call it a fire—when really, it's a line in the sand.

∾

Who made you believe walking away was failure?

Who convinced you that loyalty means staying no matter how much it hurts? What did they gain by teaching you that?

_____

_____

_____

What have you tolerated in the name of "keeping the peace"?

Was it manipulation? Betrayal? Control? Criticism? Minimizing? Why did you stay? What were you hoping would change?

_____

_____

_____

Who in your life demands access to you—but doesn't offer safety, respect, or accountability in return?

Write their names. Not to shame them—but to stop protecting people who never protected you.

_____

_____

_____

What's a relationship you've been afraid to end—not because it's good, but because of how others might react?

What are you afraid they'll say about you? What do you know they'll never admit about themselves?

_____

_____

_____

What boundaries have you set in the past that were ignored, mocked, or punished?

How did that change the way you express needs today?

_____

_____

_____

What's one boundary you've never spoken out loud, but your body has been begging you to set?

Is it space? Distance? Less contact? Total separation? Write the version that feels most honest—and most like peace.

_____

_____

_____

If you stopped trying to prove you're not the bad guy, what would you finally be free to do?

Who would you stop explaining yourself to? What would you walk away from—and never look back?

_____

_____

_____

Now Step Back and Look

People love to call it "burning bridges" when you finally stop letting them walk all over you. But a healthy boundary is not an act of destruction—it's an act of protection. If it had to be burned, maybe it was never stable to begin with.

You've tried. You've compromised. You've explained. You've prayed for change, hoped for growth, and given more chances than you had peace. And maybe you still feel guilty. That's okay. That guilt is old wiring—it was installed by people who needed your compliance to stay comfortable.

But the truth? You don't owe anyone access to you just because they once had it. You're allowed to walk away from dysfunction—even if it's family. You're allowed to stop explaining—even if they demand a story. You're allowed to protect your peace—even if it disappoints people who benefited from your pain. This isn't a grudge. It's a boundary. And it's not too late to set one.

What I grew to understand is that my boundaries had been disallowed—not ignored, not misunderstood, but flat-out disallowed. Others believed they had the right to my feelings, my reactions, my emotions. They acted as if they held the key to my survival. And for a long time, I agreed with them.

I had become captive in a life dominated by others, but also by my own fragile sense of worth, built around accept-ability. I had seen my habit of burning bridges and walking

away without a word as my cleanest escape route from pain.
I never realized I was allowed to simply say no.

No—this isn't how I see it. No—this isn't how I understand it. No—my feelings about this are different. No—I don't
like the way I'm being treated. No—what you're doing isn't
right. I know it's not right.

I saw clearly, maybe for the first time, the sacrifices I
had imposed on myself in the name of perfection. I believed
that if I could just keep up the perfect appearance, then I
would finally earn peace. But all it ever did was chain me to a
reality that wasn't mine.

This chapter stripped away the lie that walking away
was destruction. It showed me that boundaries aren't
bridges burning. They're the path back to me.

4

PRETTY HURTS & THE COST OF BEING SEEN

NAMING THE PAIN OF PERFECTION

*Y*ou were told that being pretty would open doors. You were told that being desired meant you were valuable, that attention was the same as affection, and that your worth lived in someone else's eyes. And maybe you believed it—because who wouldn't want to feel chosen, seen, admired?

But no one tells you the real cost of being seen through someone else's lens. They don't tell you how often pretty turns into pressure. How beauty becomes currency. How admiration turns into expectation. How being "wanted" often means being owned.

This isn't just about how you look. It's about what you learned to believe you had to be—just to matter. Whether you were praised for your beauty or punished for not fitting in, the lie is the same: that your value is skin-deep. That if you control your appearance, maybe you can control how you're treated. That shrinking, starving, performing, or perfecting will finally keep you safe. But none of it ever really does.

This chapter is about naming the image you've been chasing—and deciding who you are without it.

~

When did you first realize your appearance affected how people treated you?

Was it praise? Was it criticism? Was it comparison? What message did you take from it—and have you ever stopped chasing it?

_____

_____

_____

What sacrifices have you made to feel beautiful, accepted, or admired?

Think about time, money, health, dignity, silence. What have you endured in the name of looking the part?

_____

_____

_____

What do you believe you have to *look like* in order to feel lovable or worthy?

Be honest. Thin enough? Youthful enough? Flawless enough? Who taught you those requirements?

_____

_____

_____

Have you ever used your appearance as protection or power?

What did it give you? What did it cost? Did you feel empowered—or exposed?

_____

_____

_____

What emotions do you feel when you look in the mirror today?

Is it disgust? Shame? Control? Confidence? Indifference? What does your reflection *say* to you?

_____

_____

_____

What standards are you still trying to meet that aren't even yours?

Who defined your version of beauty? Who benefits when you keep chasing it?

What part of your body or self-image have you hated—but never questioned why?

Where did that hate come from? Who put it there?

If you were never judged by your appearance again, what would change in how you show up?

What would you wear? How would you walk into a room? What would you finally stop apologizing for?

Now Step Back and Look

Pretty has never been the problem. The lie is that it's everything. They taught you to believe your power was in being seen—but never in being known. They rewarded your silence, your compliance, your appeal—but not your truth.

And maybe you internalized it. Maybe you built an identity around being desired because it was safer than being dismissed. But attention is not love. Approval is not belonging. And starving yourself for someone else's definition of beauty will never fill the hunger to be accepted as you are.

You are not an ornament. You are not a product. You are not a reflection of someone else's fantasy. You are more than how you're seen. And you've always been worth more than what they told you beauty would buy.

It's time to let go of the performance. To stand in the mirror without asking for permission to love what you see. To stop trying to earn safety with a smile. This isn't about giving up. It's about getting free.

> *I learned early that my looks had value, that my figure had prestige, and that my personal mirror to the world needed to be perfect—polished, alert, and always ready to please. I always had to play the role: cute and smiling, bubbly and enthusiastic, controlled and sought after, desired, pleasing.*

This image allowed me to be seen—but it never allowed me to be known.

It taught me to be quiet. Or quieter than most of the others, but still not expected to outperform anyone. I had learned to earn safety through a smile, to perform for expectations, desires, and rules that were never mine but always required. And I chased pretty for most of my life without even knowing I was in the race.

5

MOTHERHOOD IS NOT A HALLMARK CARD

LOVE THAT DOESNT HAVE TO BE ACKNOWLEDGED

*T*hey don't write greeting cards for this. Not for the mother who did her best and still got erased. Not for the parent who stayed—who showed up, who sacrificed—and ended up cut off. There's no gold-foil sympathy for the kind of grief that comes when your child is still alive but gone. People don't talk about this kind of abandonment because it doesn't fit the script. We're told that mothers are supposed to love unconditionally. That love always wins.

That if you just keep reaching out, they'll come around. But what happens when they don't?

What happens when the child you raised writes you out of the story? When the phone goes quiet, the holidays pass, the blame gets louder, and the silence gets heavier? You grieve—and you start to question everything. Was I too much? Was I not enough? Did I fail? Or did they just choose distance because it was easier than healing?

Here's the truth no one wants to say: some children abandon their parents and rewrite the narrative to make peace with it. They'll say you were controlling, that you were emotionally unsafe, that you were never there in the way they needed. And maybe parts of that are true. Maybe you missed things. Maybe you made mistakes. All parents do.

But estrangement isn't always about truth. Sometimes, it's about power. Sometimes, they don't want healing—they want to punish you for their pain. This chapter isn't about blaming your child. It's about facing what's real—without drowning in guilt that doesn't belong to you.

ASK YOURSELF

What version of motherhood did you imagine—and what did reality look like?

Where did things go off course? Was it early on, or later in life? What do you still carry as regret, and what do you now know wasn't yours to fix?

_____

_____

_____

Have you ever been made to feel like your love didn't count because it wasn't perfect?

Who said it wasn't enough? What proof have you held on to that says otherwise?

_____

_____

_____

What have you apologized for over and over again—just to keep the door cracked open?

Have your apologies brought peace? Or just delayed your grief?

What was stolen from you in the role of being "Mom"?

Was it identity? Freedom? Safety? Your voice? How much of yourself did you give away hoping for love in return?

How have others judged your parenting without knowing the full story?

What assumptions did they make? What did they never see behind closed doors?

What would you say to the child who walked away—if you knew they would never respond?

Write it. Not to change them. To release it.

_____

_____

_____

What would peace look like if it didn't require reunion or approval?

If they never apologized. If they never returned. If they never gave you closure. What would it mean to be free anyway?

_____

_____

_____

Now Step Back and Look

You loved. You tried. You gave everything you had—sometimes more than you could afford. Maybe you yelled. Maybe you broke down. Maybe you held it all together with shaking hands. But you showed up.

And now you're standing in the wreckage of what didn't go right, trying to find peace without pretending. Here's what you need to know: you can grieve without hating. You can let go without blaming. You can choose peace without rewriting the truth.

You don't need to prove your love. You don't need to perform for forgiveness. You don't need to carry shame for someone else's choice to leave. If they come back one day, let it be because of truth—not guilt. And if they don't, let it be because your healing mattered more than waiting.

This isn't the motherhood they sell on cards. It's not soft or sparkly or tied with a bow. It's blood, loss, grit, and surrender. But there is still beauty here—in the clarity, in the release, in the quiet dignity of knowing you didn't quit on them, and you didn't quit on yourself. This is what real love looks like when it has nothing left to prove.

I had to be brave enough to write it all down. I had to be bold enough to say the truth no one ever wanted to be said. I had to be brave enough to expose a lifetime of shame.
Rejection was a wound from childhood, one I've carried since my earliest comprehension. Not being enough. Always

failing to expectations. Sacrificing my own emotional health to appease others. Realizing that motherhood should have been the absolute hallmark of my life—and realizing it was my greatest disappointment—was humbling.

I had a deep desire to love with an even deeper need to be loved back, unconditionally, completely, and with respect. When I realized that was not to be my path, I had to make peace with it. I had to see out of the fog that kept me trapped in a cycle of emotional abuse for years. I had to realize that love is not enough, and that abusive strongholds had to stop.

I learned that healing can grow even in the silence, and that forgiveness is the greatest gift Christ gives to us. I had to accept that my well-being couldn't stay at the bottom of my list. I had to prioritize myself. I had to break free from the shame and guilt imposed on me.

And in that process, I found peace in the absence and strength in the silence. I came out stronger.

6

BEHIND CLOSED DOORS

RAPE, DOMESTIC ABUSE, AND WHEN SEXUALITY BECOMES A WEAPON

Content Warning — Sexual Violence.
This chapter contains references to rape, incest, and self-seeking sexual abuse. Go slowly and ground yourself as needed. If you feel overwhelmed, step away and return when you're ready. If you are currently in crisis, please reach out for help. In the U.S., call or text 988 for the Suicide & Crisis Lifeline. If you are in immediate danger, dial 911 or your local emergency number. For support related to sexual violence, you can also call RAINN's National Sexual Assault Hotline at 1-800-656-4673. You are not alone.

a buse doesn't always take the same shape. Sometimes it's a partner who forces you. Sometimes it's a stranger who corners you. Sometimes it's family who violates you. Maybe it's you who are abusing yourself. But no matter who it is, the damage cuts deep because sexuality was meant to be connection, intimacy, and trust; instead, it became violence, control, and theft. The trauma of sexual abuse is far more widespread than most people will admit. It hides behind closed doors, inside families, inside marriages, and within the silence of survivors who were told to keep quiet. Statistics claim one in three women and one in six men will experience it in some form, but numbers can't capture the truth: every violation rewires a life. This chapter is not about statistics. It's about the reality that abuse is not rare, not "out there," and not only someone else's story. It's here. It's everywhere. And it must be named.

This chapter is not about preserving reputations. It's about calling it what it was: the rape, the betrayal, the silence that followed, and the way your own sexuality was turned against you. Take a breath and move slowly—give yourself the space to feel safe enough to name your predators. Allow yourself to acknowledge how you were abused in ways that altered the course of your life. Give yourself permission to recognize, with clarity, that you were never to blame.

~

Ask Yourself

When did your partner or spouse force themselves on you?

Write the moment without softening it. What words did they use to excuse it—"You're my wife," "It's no big deal," "This is your duty"? Write them exactly.

_____

_____

_____

Which family member raped you?

Write their name and don't protect them here; if this wasn't in your life, write the name of someone you know who was a victim of incest. How did your family's silence or denial protect the abuser instead of you— did you tell, or did you bury it so deep you forgot it was there?

_____

_____

_____

What message did your sexual attack tattoo on your body or your mind about who you are?

How have you punished yourself with your own body—through sex, denial, or shame—to numb the feelings of the past?

_____

_____

_____

Who have you slept with not out of desire, but out of fear, loneliness, or the need to feel wanted or powerful?

Write their name(s).

_____

_____

_____

What do you use sex to cover up, control, or escape in your life today?

Write this sentence: "I betrayed myself by using my body to _____ because I thought _____."

_____

_____

_____

If your body could speak honestly about your choices, what would it say back to you?

_____

_____

_____

Now Step Back and Look

It's not enough to admit what happened; you have to admit what it did to you. Trauma doesn't stay behind in the moment— it leaks into everything, into whom you trust, who you sleep with, into what you let people call love, into the way you punish your body, into the choices you make just to feel wanted. Now you step forward by tracing how violation shaped your actions. How many times did you say yes when everything in you was screaming no? Can you set a boundary that no one will ever touch you again without your consent? How many partners did you choose not out of desire, but because you were trying to erase what happened? When did sex become a transaction—a way to buy safety, attention, or control? How did shame dictate the way you walked into rooms, the way you dressed, the way you let people touch you? How often have you betrayed yourself because of what someone else did to you?

This is where you write it: every pattern, every time you repeated the wound, every place where their crime bled into your choices. Because stepping forward isn't pretending you've "moved on." It's dragging the full cost of trauma into the light so you can finally stop living like it owns you. You are loved. You are whole. You don't have to wear the marks that were imposed upon you anymore. It's called freedom once you let the light in. You will never be the same once you truly release their shame that you have been carrying.

Now step Forward

Read what you just wrote. Don't skim it. Don't minimize it. Sit in the truth of what's on these pages. You may have admitted for the first time who raped you. You may have confessed how many times you've given your body away hoping to erase the pain. You may have written the words you swore you'd never say out loud. This is not weakness. This is exposure. And exposure is the beginning of freedom. Behind closed doors, they tried to control you. They tried to silence you. They tried to bury you in shame. But here, in black and white, you just dragged it into the light. Don't look away now. This is the point where you stop carrying their crime as your identity.

My sexual trauma started early—so early, in fact, that I didn't have the name, the words, or the emotional intelligence to even understand what had happened to me. I just pushed it down deep and ran away from my pain. I didn't know I could tell. I didn't have anyone to tell and still be safe. My predator was the one who made me feel safe. He said he loved me, and I was naïve enough to believe him. I willingly kept him in my life, even knowing he had discarded my body, my morals, and broken my identity as a woman. I just wanted to be loved.

When I was assaulted at sixteen, I became broken. The rage against me changed the course of my life. I became disposable. I believed myself worthless. As I got older, I turned into a predator myself. It became a game of power and control. It was a rush to get men to go back to my room and sleep with me. There were so many that I lost names, lost cities, and certainly lost the memories because they were all hollow and empty. I betrayed myself—using my body to feed my need for validation and power because I thought I was unworthy of love. My abuse of my own body became a transactional need just to be fed. I felt I deserved this. I told myself I was in charge. I played into this destructive mindset until I was in my late forties.

But stepping out of my own game of destructive intimacy

wasn't enough. I had to face it all. I had to name it. I had to feel it. To heal, I used EMDR and ART therapies to release my inner child and comfort her pain. Complex trauma works to keep memories tucked away to keep you safe. It's a survival skill. Only once I began unleashing these memories in a healthy mindset through therapy could I understand the extent of the damage that childhood trauma had over my life. For the first time, I could truly see my past for what it was— a blessing that I survived. As I picked the stories that would go into my book about my abuse, I realized how much I had healed. I had finally laid down my greatest shame: denial. Healing became possible when I stopped lying to myself.

7

WAS IT LOVE OR JUST LOYALTY?

RELEASING THE MIND GAMES OF GUILT

*B*reaking trauma bonds, codependency, and the myths we mistake for love begins with this: sometimes the person you can't let go of is the very person who taught you that love feels like pain. They didn't have to hit you. They just had to keep you guessing—hot one minute, cold the next. Attentive when they needed you, distant when you needed them.

So you learned to stay. To serve. To fix. To sacrifice. To carry the relationship on your back—because walking away felt like betrayal. But love isn't supposed to feel like punishment. And loyalty doesn't mean abandoning yourself. You were trained to confuse survival with love. To call control "care." To call anxiety "passion." To call dysfunction "chemistry." But what you called love may have just been a bond forged in fear.

This chapter isn't about shaming your past. It's about finally calling it what it was—so you don't keep repeating it.

~

Ask Yourself

Who made you feel responsible for their emotions, reactions, or healing?

Did they praise your empathy but punish your boundaries? How did they hook you—and what did they make you afraid to lose?

_____

_____

_____

What relationships in your life felt intense but unsafe?

Did you feel addicted to them? Couldn't let go even when it hurt? What did you mistake for "love" in that dynamic?

_____

_____

_____

When did you start believing your value came from being needed?

Who rewarded you for showing up small, silent, or selfless? Who made your identity about what you could _give_?

_____

_____

_____

What patterns do you keep repeating in relationships—romantic, familial, or even friendships?

Are you the fixer? The one who absorbs? The one who disappears? The one who chases?

_____

_____

_____

What myths about love have shaped your decisions?

That love is sacrifice? That love requires pain? That walking away means failure? Where did those beliefs come from?

_____

_____

_____

Who have you stayed loyal to—long after they stopped being loyal to you?

Write their name. Don't justify it. Just be honest about the imbalance.

_____

_____

_____

What parts of yourself have you betrayed in the name of "being good" or "staying connected"?

Your voice? Your body? Your boundaries? Your dreams?

_____

_____

_____

Now Step Back and Look

There's a reason it was hard to leave. Trauma bonds feel like love when pain is all you've known. Codependency feels like connection when your worth has always been measured by how much you give. You weren't weak for staying. You were conditioned. You were loyal. You were hopeful.

But now you see it: love doesn't require you to disappear. Loyalty doesn't mean lifelong suffering. And commitment doesn't mean abandoning your own truth. Some people will call it "giving up" when you finally let go. But deep down, you know what it is. It's clarity. It's healing. It's love—real love—starting with yourself.

You don't need to rewrite the past. You just need to stop repeating it. Break the bond. Cut the cord. Tell the truth. Choose peace—even if no one claps for it. This time, let love look like safety. Let loyalty look like honesty. Let healing look like walking away when the price is you.

I wrote through the stories of the love I held for my family, my husbands, and my friends that wasn't returned. I had protected myself by believing their love was genuine—that they truly liked what they saw underneath my surface, and that they genuinely held loyalty toward me. I was deceived.

I learned that I had to put others in front of myself daily, weekly, hourly. People-pleasing, going over the top, and being an overachiever was where I felt the safest. If I could supply something—anything or everything—for someone else, that became the very thing they expected from me. And boy, did they take.

I stayed too long in relationships that had run their course. In relationships that had grown accustomed to taking and never giving anything back. I stayed too long in many of these relationships because I had not yet found my voice. All I heard was their voice of demands.

And then I chose me.

8

FREEZE. FAWN. FLIGHT. FIGHT.

UNDERSTANDING TRAUMA RESPONSES AND THE PATTERNS THAT PROTECT US

*Y*ou didn't choose this. You didn't sit down and decide to freeze when the pressure rose. You didn't plan to people-please. You didn't want to run from connection or explode in defense. These weren't conscious choices. These were instincts, wired into your nervous system the moment your body realized the world was not safe. Freeze. Fawn. Flight. Fight. Four trauma responses. Four ways you learned to survive. And that is the reason you still feel exhausted, over-reactive, numb, avoidant, overly accommodating—or like you're always on edge. This chapter is not about judgment. It's about recognition. Because once you name your pattern, you can stop being ruled by it.

FREEZE

The world becomes too much. Your brain slows. You go blank. You don't cry. You don't scream. You check out. Not because you don't care —but because your body shuts down before the pain can register. Freeze looks like brain fog during conflict, emotional numbness, inability to make decisions, withdrawing when overwhelmed, and "shutting down" in high-stress environments. It was never laziness. It was the only way to feel safe when escape wasn't an option.

FAWN

You avoid conflict at all costs. You become who others want you to be. You apologize for things that weren't your fault. You keep the peace—even when it means betraying yourself. Fawn looks like people-pleasing to the point of burnout, constant self-editing, feeling responsible for others' emotions, saying "yes" when you want to say "no," and feeling anxious if someone is mad at you. Fawning kept you from being hurt. But now it keeps you from being seen.

FLIGHT

You don't deal—you do. You stay busy. Productive. Focused. Anything to avoid the stillness where the pain lives. Flight looks like obsessive planning, workaholism, avoiding intimacy, always needing a distraction, and constant movement to outrun the past. Flight told you that if you just keep going, the pain can't catch you. But healing doesn't happen at full speed.

FIGHT

You lash out. You snap. You control. Not because you're cruel, but because your nervous system is in full alarm mode. You learned that attack is the best defense. Fight looks like a quick temper, needing to win arguments, controlling people or outcomes, reacting before thinking, and righteous anger that isolates you. You weren't trying to destroy connection—you were trying to protect yourself from being destroyed again.

These Aren't Just Reactions. They're Survival Blueprints

Your body didn't betray you. It kept you alive. But here's the truth: what protected you then may be harming you now. Not because you're broken, but because you're safe now—and your nervous system hasn't caught up yet. That's not your fault. But it is your responsibility to start healing it.

∼

Which trauma response shows up most often in your life today?

What does it look like in your relationships, career, parenting, or faith?

_____

_____

_____

When did you first learn that response?

Go back. What was happening around you? Who were you trying to please, escape, defend against, or survive?

_____

_____

_____

What did that response protect you from?

What would have happened if you had spoken up? Said no? Asked for what you needed?

_____

_____

_____

Where does that response still serve you—and where does it limit your freedom?

How has it shaped your identity, and how does it keep you from showing up as your full self?

_____

_____

_____

What would it feel like to respond from choice instead of reflex?

What might you say, do, or feel if you weren't stuck in the past?

_____

_____

_____

What does your body need to feel safe again?

Not to perform safety—but to *embody* it? Name one practice, boundary, or truth that helps.

_____

_____

_____

Now Step Back and Look

You're not crazy. You're not too sensitive. You're not unstable or dramatic. You are a trauma survivor with a brilliant, sensitive nervous system that adapted in ways no one else could see. And while the world may judge the outward response, only you know the war you've fought internally just to exist. You froze to keep from being punished. You fawned to avoid being left. You fled to outrun the chaos. You fought to protect what was left of you. You survived. But now, you get to live.

That means slowing down, noticing your body, naming your patterns, and choosing differently—not because you were wrong, but because you're finally safe enough to do it another way. This isn't about eliminating your trauma responses. It's about honoring them—and no longer letting them run the show. Your brain did its job. Now it's time to teach it that you're home.

With my ongoing therapy and exploration, when childhood complex trauma begins to evade and interrupt my thinking, I've had to clearly understand the four trauma markers: Freeze. Fawn. Flight. Fight. In the stories I uncovered and shared with the world, all four of these trauma markers were playing in my heart, mind, and soul—and they were clearly in charge. For me, they were interchangeable. Stay alert to trickery. Stay ahead. Smile. Appease. Run. Shut down.

Learning to people-please at such a young age, at the

hand of my mother and inside my intimate family circle, taught me how to fawn. Experiencing sexual abuse at such a young age heightened my freeze response. My body learned quickly that stillness was safer than risk. My flight response? That was masterful. I was born with the need to get away—to keep moving, not stay long enough to be tracked, and be ready to leave the meeting, the relationship, the room without notice. Be ready to run.

Fight—that instinct came later than I would've expected. Sure, I can be a fighter. But for so many years, I never raised my sword. I just knelt deep and asked, "How much more, sir?" None of these trauma responses are bad. They're signals. They're internal alerts letting your psyche know: "Something is very wrong." But when you start living through them—using them as your operating system just to get through the day, the hour, the moment—then it's time to have a very serious conversation with yourself. This isn't just about awareness. It's about rescue.

Out of all the workbook pages, this one deserves your full attention. These four trauma responses can distort your perception of self. They can cloud your judgment. They can twist your understanding of other people's intentions. If you want to find your footing again, start here. Because survival is not your identity—and you were never meant to live your life in constant reaction.

9

I STAYED—BUT WHY?

THE RELIEF OF TAKING ACCOUNTABILITY

*T*his chapter is for the one who keeps asking, why did I stay, and finally deserves the real answer.

Understanding abuse, addiction to chaos, and the illusion of control means facing the question the world never stops asking: Why didn't you leave? Why did you go back? Why did you stay so long?—as if survival were ever that tidy, as if a clean escape were the only story worth telling. You stayed because you believed you could fix it, because it was good once and maybe it could be again, because you were trauma-bonded, confused, afraid, and isolated, because your nervous system had been trained to find familiarity in dysfunction, because the moment you tried to leave the person hurting you became the person begging you to stay. And for a while, that chaos felt like love—the highs euphoric, the lows annihilating—until safety became something you measured by how well you could manage the explosion, whispering to yourself, If I just do this differently, maybe he won't get angry. If I'm quieter, more understanding, less myself. Yet that was never love—only control disguised as chemistry, addiction disguised as devotion, abuse rewriting itself in your mind as you're overreacting.

Ask Yourself

What did you believe would change if you just held on a little longer?

What did they promise you? What did you keep hoping for? What pieces of good did you use to excuse the bad?

_____

_____

_____

How were you made to feel like the abuse was your fault?

Were you called crazy? Too sensitive? Overdramatic? What tactics did they use to make you question your reality?

_____

_____

_____

When did the cycle start to feel normal—even comforting?

What moments of calm made you second-guess leaving? Did you start to feel powerful when you could predict their moods?

_____

_____

_____

What part of you believed you could save them?

Where did that belief come from—childhood, faith, desperation, pride? What did you sacrifice trying to redeem someone who never wanted to change?

_____

_____

_____

Did you ever feel addicted to the chaos—even as it destroyed you?

Be honest. Did the silence feel worse than the storm? Did you mistake intensity for intimacy?

_____

_____

_____

What "control" did you think you had?

Were you managing the moods, the house, the conversation, the story? What were you really trying to keep from falling apart?

_____

_____

_____

What finally made you leave—or what still keeps you tied to them?

If you left, what was the breaking point? If you stayed, what are you still afraid of?

_____

_____

_____

Now Step Back and Look

You didn't stay because you were stupid. You stayed because you were surviving, because you believed what they told you, because somewhere along the way love had been rewired into endurance. You kept the peace, you made excuses, you hid the bruises—emotional or physical—and you told yourself it wasn't that bad, told others you were fine, while the truth was you were drowning in a relationship where love was a leash and survival was called strength.

It's okay to admit it now: it wasn't love, it wasn't safe, it wasn't you. Let go of the illusion that if you had just done something differently it would have worked, let go of the need to explain your choices to people who never lived through your silence, let go of the guilt for not leaving sooner, let go of the shame for how long you stayed. You are not weak for being loyal; you are strong for telling the truth now. Healing begins the moment you stop rewriting the past and start reclaiming your voice. You stayed—but now you see it, and that's where the freedom begins.

The illusion of control had taken over my entire identity. I had a role, a purpose, and a drive to succeed that was unquenchable. But every day I stayed I worked, I slaved, I excelled, and still I was failing, because underneath I had become addicted to the chaos. Over time, I began to understand that I had also become addicted to the abuse itself, to the cycle that kept me running faster, harder, longer, as though by sheer effort I could prove something—my worth, my lovability, my commitment. Trauma doesn't care about logic; it traps you in patterns and cycles of destruction so well disguised that you don't even know you've fallen into them.

Because I saw myself as competent and powerful, I believed I could fix anything, anyone, and if I was still succeeding then nothing could truly be wrong. I convinced myself that trying harder would eventually make it all work. But that was the lie—the loop—that kept me locked, frozen in circumstances that were slowly killing me.

PART II

Breaking Points

Survival only works for so long. Eventually the cracks show, the body buckles, the truth bleeds through. Breaking points don't come to destroy you — they come to reveal what silence and shame have been covering. Grief, pain, depression, anger, addiction, imposter syndrome — these are the places where life demanded honesty. In this Stage, you'll name the moments you said, "I can't keep carrying this." Because naming your breaking point is the first step toward refusing to live broken.

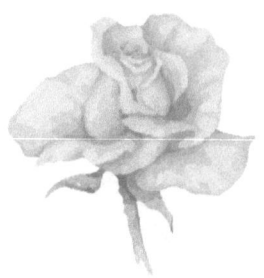

10

DRESSED FOR THE JOB— BLEEDING ON THE INSIDE

WORKPLACE DYSFUNCTION, PROFESSIONALISM UNDER PRESSURE, AND THE MASKS WE WEAR

*Y*ou walk in polished, composed, and prepared—your résumé clean, your posture straight, your voice measured—yet behind the blazer your heart is racing, behind the smile a scream is swallowed, and behind the performance there is a person who feels like she's dying inside and either no one sees it or, worse, someone does and weaponizes it; welcome to workplace dysfunction, where speaking up is labeled "abrasive," where boundaries are translated as "not a team player," where excellence is expected but confidence is punished, and where you're told to "bring your whole self to work" until your whole self makes someone uncomfortable.

This chapter is written for the ones who kept it together in the meeting and fell apart in the bathroom stall, for the ones who were branded "difficult" for noticing the truth, for the ones who outperformed and outlasted yet were still outcast; you weren't crazy, you weren't overreacting—you were bleeding in a place that only rewarded silence.

~

Ask Yourself

Have you ever been praised for your professionalism—while silently suffering?

What did you hide to keep your job, your image, or your sanity intact? What did it cost you?

_____

_____

_____

When did you start believing that your worth depended on being the most competent, least emotional person in the room?

Who taught you that feelings are dangerous? Who rewarded your performance—but ignored your pain?

_____

_____

_____

What workplace dynamics have made you question your reality?

Were you gaslit? Undermined? Excluded? What did they make you believe about *yourself*?

_____

_____

_____

What labels were you given for simply standing your ground?

Were you called intimidating? Emotional? Angry? Aggressive? Uncoachable? Unprofessional? How did those words shape your behavior?

_____

_____

_____

Have you ever had to choose between being liked and being honest?

What did you say—or stay silent about—to keep the peace? How did that peace feel in your body?

_____

_____

_____

What role do you play at work that doesn't align with who you really are?

The fixer? The silent one? The people-pleaser? The perfectionist? What would happen if you dropped the mask?

_____

_____

_____

If you were completely safe to tell the truth at work, what would you say—and to whom?

Write the unspoken. Even if you never say it out loud, say it *here*.

_____

_____

_____

Now Step Back and Look

It wasn't only the job that broke you, it was the culture that told you your instincts were wrong, the systems that rewarded manipulation and punished truth, the environments that renamed dysfunction "leadership" and called control "collaboration." You adapted: you toned it down, you stayed late, you delivered results—and still they made you the problem; but here's what's real: you were never too much, you were a mirror, and mirrors make people uncomfortable when they're not ready to see the cracks. The pressure to stay quiet was not professionalism but self-erasure; the praise for holding it together was not admiration but exploitation; the job title didn't protect you and the paycheck didn't validate you—yes, you did the work, but they drained your spirit.

It is not weakness to say it hurt; it is not bitterness to name what they did; it is not disloyalty to want better. This is how you stop bleeding: call out the cut, take off the mask, and decide that dignity is worth more than being tolerated. You can be excellent and exhausted, honest and professional, walk away and still hold your head high; this isn't quitting, it's reclaiming your power.

In my own story I traced the same pattern I had learned in childhood into the fluorescent hallways of corporate life—stay small, be agreeable, and for God's sake be nice —so I performed, wearing the clothes, holding the meetings, making the sales, setting the bar and driving for more every single day against myself until I raised my voice and my voice was crushed and, suddenly, I became the problem. I learned I wasn't liked, wasn't expected to last, and still wasn't good enough—until I said, "no more," reclaimed my voice, and reclaimed the right to be me.

11

WHEN THE STRONG ONE BREAKS

COMPLEX PTSD, EMOTIONAL COLLAPSE, AND THE BREAKING POINT THAT SAVES YOU

*Y*ou were the one who held it together—the dependable one, the one who didn't cry, didn't crack, didn't crumble. You got the job done, you raised the kids, you smiled through the meetings. You were the strong one—until you weren't.

Because even strength has a breaking point. And when it hits, it doesn't always look like a dramatic scene; sometimes it looks like silence, exhaustion, brain fog, emotional shutdown, chronic illness, or standing in the kitchen, staring at a dark window, and wondering how you got there.

This chapter isn't about weakness. It's about Complex PTSD—and what happens when survival mode finally runs out of fuel.

WHAT IS COMPLEX PTSD (CPTSD)?

Unlike acute trauma, which comes from a single terrifying event, Complex PTSD develops from chronic, repeated trauma over time— especially during formative years or within relationships where escape was not possible.

CPTSD often forms in emotionally abusive or neglectful households, long-term relationships with narcissists, addicts, or manipulators, high-control environments such as workplaces or religious settings, or situations where you had to suppress your needs just to stay "safe." And here's the part most people miss: people with CPTSD usually look high-functioning—until they don't.

Common Signs You're the "Strong One" with CPTSD

You minimize your own pain, telling yourself that "other people have it worse." You numb out in high-stress moments but crash later. You fear being a burden, so you isolate instead. You're hyper-independent but secretly exhausted. You over-perform at work but feel emotionally hollow. You can't rest—even when you try. You don't trust safety, so you sabotage it. You don't cry when you should, but you collapse when no one sees.

Sound familiar? That's not personality. That's programming. And when the system finally overloads, you break.

But here's the shift: that breaking point isn't the end—it's the beginning. It's where the mask falls off, where survival stops working, where real healing can finally start.

~

ASK YOURSELF

What does your body do when you're overwhelmed—but trying to hold it together?

Do you clench? Shake? Numb out? Dissociate? Shut down emotionally? Describe it.

_____

_____

_____

When did "being strong" become your identity—and what were you protecting?

Who needed you to stay strong for them? What did falling apart feel like it would cost you?

_____

_____

_____

What was your moment of collapse?

Was it slow or sudden? Public or private? What triggered it—and what truth did it reveal?

_____

_____

_____

What reactions did you get when you finally broke?

Did people show up for you? Or did they walk away? Did they minimize it? Did anyone call it brave?

_____

_____

_____

What would it look like to allow your nervous system to rest without guilt?

What would rest *feel* like in your body? What are you afraid will happen if you slow down?

_____

_____

_____

What does your strength look like now that you know the difference between surviving and healing?

What traits still serve you? What coping mechanisms can you release?

_____

_____

_____

Now Step Back and Look

The strong one isn't the one who never breaks; the strong one is the one who dares to fall apart—and still gets back up. Your collapse was never weakness. It was the wisdom of your body screaming: No more. No more pretending. No more people-pleasing. No more emotional suppression dressed up as resilience.

This is the point where your nervous system stops fighting and starts healing. Where you stop proving your worth through suffering. Where you stop calling your trauma "personality." This is where the unraveling becomes sacred.

You are allowed to be exhausted. You are allowed to cry. You are allowed to need. You are allowed to stop performing strength and start receiving rest. The world may not applaud your breakdown—but heaven sees it as the start of your rebuild.

When my life patterns had become so guttural, so deep, and the pain of keeping it all together had become immeasurable, I broke. And I didn't just break a little. I crawled out of hell on my hands and knees, over glass and coals, just to start the path to healing.

I was force-fed the realization that I had complex childhood trauma—Complex PTSD—the result of how I had been raised and conditioned since birth. Psychological abuse had been perpetuated against me in young adulthood and followed me all the way into my corporate life.

I learned that I had been overachieving, dissociating, and numbing—all while fighting the daily fear of abandonment and the fear of losing my relevance if I didn't perform. I learned that my nervous system had endured years of staying on high alert to ensure everyone else's needs were met —and now, I was unraveling.

My persistence had gotten me this far. But it came at an extreme cost to my health.

IMPOSTER SYNDROME WASN'T LYING—BUT IT WASN'T RIGHT EITHER

RECLAIMING YOUR WORTH IN THE FACE OF INNER CRITICS.

*Y*ou didn't just wake up one day thinking you were a fraud. That belief was built—layer by layer—by environments that told you that you were either too much or not enough. Maybe it was teachers. Or parents. Or employers. Maybe it was being the only one like you in the room—and being reminded of it. Maybe it was being praised for performance, but punished for presence. Or maybe it was simply Complex PTSD doing what it does best: whispering self-doubt in your strongest moments.

Imposter syndrome doesn't always mean you're wrong about yourself. Sometimes, it means you were trained to believe that your instincts were invalid, your voice too loud, your brilliance suspicious. So yes, the voice in your head might sound like the truth. But that doesn't mean it's right.

WHAT IMPOSTER SYNDROME OFTEN SOUNDS LIKE

"I don't belong here."
"I must've fooled them."
"I'm not qualified enough."
"They're going to find out I'm not really that good."
"If I slow down, I'll be exposed."

"Success just means higher risk of failure."

And if you have Complex PTSD, those thoughts aren't random—they're rooted in long-term exposure to invalidation, emotional neglect, and gaslighting. You were taught not to trust yourself. So it makes perfect sense that when you finally succeed... you question everything.

ASK YOURSELF

When did you first feel like you had to prove your worth just to belong?

Was it school? Family? Work? What were the stakes if you didn't outperform?

_____

_____

_____

What spaces made you question your intelligence, value, or capability?

Did someone else get the credit? Did you shrink back? Did you mask confidence while secretly spiraling?

_____

_____

_____

What role did perfectionism play in your survival?

Did you believe mistakes made you unlovable? Were you praised for being "resilient" when you were really just scared?

What kind of feedback triggers your imposter voice the loudest?

Praise? Criticism? Silence? Who do you still hear in your head when you doubt yourself?

Have you ever accomplished something and felt nothing?

Did success feel dangerous, temporary, or unearned? What did you immediately pressure yourself to do next?

What story do you tell yourself about what kind of person deserves to be seen, heard, and trusted?

Does that person look like you? Sound like you? Or have you excluded yourself from your own standard?

_____

_____

_____

If you stopped striving to earn belonging, what would you finally be free to own?

Write down what is already true about your value—even if you don't feel it yet.

_____

_____

_____

Now Step Back and Look

Imposter syndrome isn't just insecurity—it's evidence. Evidence that somewhere along the line, you were made to feel small on purpose. That someone benefited from your silence. That institutions capitalized on your second-guessing. That whole systems were built to make you question your seat at the table.

So when that voice creeps in again—the one that says you're not enough—don't just argue with it. Interrogate it. Where did it come from? Who does it sound like? What does it want you to shrink for?

You're not a fraud for feeling like an outsider. You're a survivor of spaces that were never designed for you to thrive. But you're here. You didn't fake it. You fought for it. And you don't have to keep apologizing for what you've earned just because someone else is uncomfortable.

> With this realization, I had to take a painfully hard look at myself and try to understand who I really am. By this point, I had no idea. I had always been too much. Too bossy. Too this. Too that. These flaws I had been programmed to believe my whole life ran like a loop in my head. I felt the need to shrink myself down—and that feeling had been reinforced through childhood. Stay small. Stay silent. Don't expect much. And whatever you do—don't outshine.
>
> I realized I had been living in a lie. I had relied on others' judgment and criticism to shape the value of my iden-

tity. And I felt I had to perform to keep it. The woman I had become? I was an expert imposter.

As my writing became clearer, I had to expose it all. Not just the stories that were acceptable. Not just the stories that left a good feeling in your gut. The truth had to come out—and it had to come out exactly what it was: the truth of my situation in the current. Not through rose-colored glasses.

I had to reclaim my worth. I had to reclaim my identity. I had to expose myself to heal.

As all the stories started tumbling out of me, I wrote each one in great graphic detail. But once the manuscript was completed, I had to begin the ominous task of editing. Editing was difficult. Which words to leave in. Which words to leave out. How much do you share? How much do you keep behind the curtain? How much do you save for fear that no one would actually understand?

This impostor—she had to go.

1 3

GRIEVING THE LIFE YOU DIDN'T GET (AMBIGUOUS LOSS)

NAMING THE FUNERALS WE NEVER GET— SO ANGER CAN BECOME CLARITY, NOT CHAOS

*Y*ou can't mourn what you were never allowed to name. There was no casket, no service, no casseroles—just a quiet ache for the parent you needed, the childhood you deserved, the family that never became safe. This is ambiguous loss: grief that doesn't end because it never got to begin. They're still alive, or the story never started, and yet something real died—the future you were promised, the comfort you were owed, the love that never learned how. People tell you to be grateful, to let it go, to move on. But you can't bury what no one admits has passed, so it follows you—birthday after birthday, holiday after holiday—a shadow at the table where safety should have sat. This chapter is permission to say what was missing, to honor what never arrived, to mark the losses that shaped you so they stop ruling you from the dark.

Ambiguous loss often feels like invisible grief with no ritual and no witness; hope looping with dread ("maybe this year will be different"); being triggered by "normal" moments—photos, holidays, milestones; self-blame for wanting what should have been basic; anger that turns inward because there's nowhere else to place it; numbness that suddenly cracks into floods of tears you can't explain; the ache of being an adult who still needed a safe lap. This isn't drama—it's mourning without a map. And you're allowed to grieve the mother or father you needed but didn't have; the apology you deserved and never got; the sibling or child who chose the family myth over the truth; the home that required performance to be allowed inside; the church that protected image over people; the mentor who saw your brilliance and used it instead of blessing it; the birthdays you pretended were fine; the version of you who never had to be on guard. You don't owe anyone a sanitized eulogy for what hurt you.

~

Ask Yourself

What didn't you receive that you still ache for?

Name it without shrinking—safety, presence, protection, delight. Choose the exact words.

_____

_____

_____

What ritual would honor that loss?

A letter you won't send, lighting a candle on a meaningful date, planting a tree, marking an empty chair and praying a lament.

_____

_____

_____

Where did you learn to minimize your grief so others stayed comfortable?

Who taught you your longing was "too much," and how did that shape your voice?

What timeline did you build around someone who never showed up?

How long did you wait? What did it cost you—emotionally, financially, spiritually?

What boundary will keep you from re-entering the same hope loop?

Fewer invitations, shorter calls, supervised visits, no last-minute rescues —write the line you'll hold.

If you could bless the child-you with one sentence today, what would you say?

Write it. Say it out loud. Let it land in your body.

_____

_____

_____

What memory still stings because there was no closure—and how will you close it now?

Speak it to a witness, journal it fully, take a solitary walk and release it in prayer.

_____

_____

_____

Now Step Back and Look

Grief is not blame; grief is love telling the truth about what it lost. You're not weak for wanting what was right. You're not bitter for naming what never came. You're honest. Mourning makes space—space for anger to turn into clarity instead of chaos, space for boundaries to become devotion to your nervous system rather than punishment to anyone else, space for you to stop rehearsing a rescue that isn't coming. You can bless what was real and bury what never was. You can keep your heart soft and your terms strong. You can stop waiting at the door and start setting the table for the life that actually shows up. This is not forgetting; it's finishing—so the ache can become honor, and the story can move.

> For me, I grieve the family life I never achieved. I had thought I would have the perfect family and children—happy, healthy, and full of memories and laughter. I tried. I never succeeded. I tried again. Complex generational trauma intertwined in my relationships with my children. Canceled. Silence. I failed. Or did I?
>
> I no longer have to watch my back for barbs of disapproval, or invitations that don't come. The "jokes" were always aimed at something "stupid" I said or did, and never once did anyone remember a memory the same way. I became the piggybank when they needed something, mocked and ridiculed for how bad my memory was, and the punching bag

when they felt like it. Emotional abuse and generational trauma are hard to uncover—harder still when you keep staying in the fight.

When I understood their silence was meant to punish me —and that all my tears and sadness meant nothing to them— I let it go. I let them run. I let them live their lives. Joyfully. Because that's how I am living mine. Sometimes silence is the best result when peace is the desired outcome.

14

I DIDN'T WANT TO DIE—I JUST DIDN'T WANT TO HURT ANYMORE

DEPRESSION, SUICIDAL IDEATION, AND THE PRICE OF EMOTIONAL TRAUMA PAIN

CONTENT ADVISORY — Suicidal Ideation.

This chapter discusses depression and thoughts of suicide. Please pace yourself and use the grounding tools. In the U.S., call or text 988 for the Suicide & Crisis Lifeline. If you're in immediate danger, call 911.

*Y*ou didn't write a note—or maybe you did. You didn't scream for attention; you quietly froze food for the family and organized for your departure. You didn't want people crying at your funeral; you wanted relief. Relief from waking up with a thousand pounds on your chest, from carrying the same haunting memories like weights around your ankles, from pretending you're fine while you're unraveling in silence.

This chapter isn't about pity; it's about truth—the kind of pain that doesn't show up in charts or checklists, the kind that makes death feel like peace and disappearing feel like mercy. You didn't want to die. You just didn't want to hurt anymore.

If you're here right now—pause. You don't have to carry this alone. In the U.S., call or text 988 or tell one trusted person, "I'm not okay and I need help." If you're in immediate danger, call 911.

WHAT DEPRESSION FEELS LIKE:

A fog you can't explain and can't escape.

The guilt of being tired when nothing's "wrong."

Feeling numb—but also "too much."

Shame for being ungrateful when you "have so much to live for."

Crying for help in coded trauma language and no one hearing: "I'm hurting inside." "I need help."

Thinking, "Would anyone even notice if I was gone?" "Would anyone care?" "Would I be remembered?"

Depression is not laziness. Suicidal ideation is not selfish. These are symptoms—not character flaws. And if you're reading this, you're still here. That alone is a kind of miracle.

Right Now (before you begin):

Drink a glass of water.

Open a window or step outside for one minute.

Put both feet on the floor, or melt into your favorite chair. Breathe in for 12 counts, hold for 6, and exhale until your lungs are empty. Pause for two seconds. Then inhale for 14, hold, and exhale again. Repeat this pattern 12 times. Let your body release the noise. Text someone safe: "Can you check in on me?"

≈

Ask Yourself

When did the pain start to feel louder than hope?

Was it gradual or sudden? Was there a moment you knew you were slipping?

_____

_____

_____

Who did you reach for—and who wasn't there?

Did they listen? Did they minimize? Did they turn away? How did that deepen the pain?

_____

_____

_____

What lie did depression whisper that sounded like truth?

"You're too much." "You're a burden." "You'll never be free." Which one grabbed hold of you?

_____

_____

_____

What would you say to someone else feeling how you've felt?

Say it here. Say it for them. Say it for *you*.

_____

_____

_____

What have you survived that no one else knows about?

Name it. Honor it. You're still here—and that matters more than you think.

_____

_____

_____

What's one reason you stayed—even when you didn't want to?

A name. A thought. A hope. A whisper. Write it. Don't diminish it.

_____

_____

_____

Now Step Back and Look

You weren't being dramatic or selfish; you were hurting. No one taught you how to say it out loud without fear of being labeled, medicated, or dismissed. Here's what's true: wanting the pain to stop doesn't make you broken—it makes you human.

The world doesn't know what to do with emotional pain that can't be fixed in a weekend or numbed with productivity, so you shove it down, spiritualize it, over-function, and perform healing while going quiet inside. But you weren't put here to perform; you were put here to live.

Life was never meant to feel like a punishment.

It's time to stop pretending that being alive is enough. You deserve to want to live, to feel safe in your own body, and to wake up without dreading the hours ahead.

If no one told you this before, let it land now: you are not a burden; you are not weak; you are not too far gone. Your presence matters—even on days you can't feel it. You're staying matters—even when it's quiet. Your choice to keep breathing is sacred.

This isn't about turning your story into inspiration; it's about staying in it long enough to see that the light does come back—maybe slowly, maybe in flickers, maybe with help—but it does. You didn't want to die; you just didn't want to hurt. Healing can start with that honest sentence. You're still here, and that changes everything.

Your darkest chapters weren't only filled with trauma; they carried the quiet urge to stop fighting, to leave the pain, to leave this world. Depression is real. Suicidal ideation is real. It can feel like being gagged by an invisible force—you see what's happening, but you can't stop it. Talking helps. Medication can help. Depression tells convincing lies, and you don't have to outthink it alone—help and support make the lies quieter.

Maybe you've heard it said: "Christians don't think about suicide." Maybe you were told that growing up. Maybe you heard it in church. Maybe you believed it yourself—until the day you didn't.

Because when those thoughts show up—when life feels unbearable and you wonder if it would be easier not to wake up tomorrow—that sentence doesn't sound holy anymore. It sounds like a wall. It tells you to stay quiet. It convinces you you're the only one.

But the Bible doesn't stay quiet. Elijah prayed that God would take his life. Job cursed the day he was born. Jonah told God he'd rather die than live. Paul admitted he despaired of life itself. These weren't fringe people—they were God's prophets, His chosen, His apostles. His children.

So here's the truth: Christians do think about suicide. The problem is you've been trained to hide it. You've been told it makes you faithless, when in reality it makes you human.

And the good news? God doesn't turn away. He sat with Elijah under the tree. He listened to Job rage and lament. He met Paul in his despair. He meets you, too not with judgment, but with presence.

If these thoughts visit again, make a plan: tell someone you trust, move your body for two minutes, choose one grounding prayer, and if it worsens, call or text 988 (U.S.) or emergency services if you're in immediate danger. That's not weakness. That's strength.

As I stitched my story together, I saw the bookends. My darkest chapters weren't only filled with trauma; they carried the quiet urge to stop fighting, to leave the pain, to leave this world. Depression is real. Suicidal ideation is real. It can feel like being gagged by an invisible force—you see what's happening, but you can't stop it. Talking helps. Medication can help. Depression tells convincing lies, and you don't have to outthink it alone—help and support make the lies quieter. I'd love to say I'm free of those thoughts now, but I won't lie to you. Even after all I've overcome and how far I've come, this is still something I watch for.

If your mind goes there too, hear me: you are not alone. Depression doesn't care how successful you look or whether you have a nice house or no money for milk. It doesn't care about you; it just whispers lies—"You're the problem. You're a burden. You'll never feel better." Resist those lies. There's no magic fix, but help helps—therapy, medication, community, and the love of Christ. The truth is that even when I get triggered, I now recognize the voice behind the lie, and I've learned ways to overcome.

So can you.

Depression isn't pretty, and the truth isn't pretty, but overcoming—in spite of it—is brilliant.

It's Grace.

15

NUMB UNTIL IT DESTROYS

DRUGS, ALCOHOL, AND FOOD ... — NUMBING THAT BACKFIRES

Numbing feels like relief—until it doesn't. At first, it works. The drink takes the edge off. The pill helps you sleep. The high quiets the panic in your chest. The food soothes the ache no one else sees. The shopping spree gives you a hit of control. The endless hours of work drown out what you don't want to feel. The hookup silences loneliness for a night. The scrolling and busyness keep you distracted long enough to avoid your own thoughts. You tell yourself it's manageable, that you're just taking the edge off, that everyone else does it too. For a little while, you believe it.

But numbing is never neutral. It buys silence at the expense of truth. It takes the pain down for a moment, but the cost is always higher when it comes back. Because pain that isn't healed doesn't go away—it waits. And every time you push it down with alcohol, with drugs, with food, with work, with sex, with distraction, it pushes back harder.

For survivors of trauma, numbing often starts as survival. It's not weakness. It's not rebellion. It's the body screaming, "I can't keep carrying this raw." When you have no safe place to put your pain, you find ways to dull it. And for a season, maybe it saves you. But the very thing that soothed you begins to betray you. What you thought was a lifeline becomes another chain.

Food can be one of the most deceptive forms of numbing. It doesn't come with warning labels. It doesn't raise suspicion at work or church. No one whispers behind your back about the second plate of food the way they do about a drink in your hand. Food is acceptable, even celebrated. And that makes it harder to see when it becomes a crutch.

Sometimes food numbs through restriction—controlling calories, shrinking portions, obsessing over discipline. The hunger itself becomes a distraction from emotional pain. Other times food numbs through indulgence—eating past fullness, chasing the comfort of sugar or salt, filling the emptiness inside with whatever's on the plate. Either way, food stops being nourishment and starts being anesthesia.

The truth is, trauma doesn't care whether you numb with a bottle, a pill, a binge, or a calendar packed so full you don't have a moment to feel. The cycle is the same. A feeling rises—shame, fear, loneliness, grief. You reach for what will dull it. Relief comes for a moment. Then guilt sets in. Then the shame returns heavier than before. The pattern repeats until you can't tell if you're numbing the old wound or the new one you just created.

Trauma wires the brain to expect pain, chaos, and danger. It keeps the nervous system on high alert. You don't relax—you scan. You don't rest —you brace. Your body is flooded with cortisol and adrenaline, always ready to fight, flee, freeze, or fawn. Numbing interrupts that flood, even if only for a few hours. It tells the body, "Stand down." It quiets the alarm bells that never stop ringing.

But here's the truth: numbing doesn't just shut off pain. It also shuts off joy. It blunts the panic, but it blunts peace too. It buries shame, but it buries love too. You stop feeling the terror, but you stop feeling alive. Over time, you forget what it means to live without a chemical filter, a full plate, a crowded schedule, or a false intimacy. You start believing you can't.

You numb because trauma trained you to survive, not to feel. You numb because your story told you feelings were dangerous—that crying made you weak, that anger would get you punished, that joy was fleeting, that sadness made you a burden. You numb because silence was safer than honesty, and numbing was easier than chaos.

But the truth is this: you never numbed because you wanted to destroy yourself. You numbed because you wanted to save yourself. And you did —for a while. But survival has an expiration date. What once saved you is now killing you.

When did you first use alcohol or drugs to make the pain go quiet?

Write down the memory. What were you escaping?

_____

_____

_____

What did the substance give you that you couldn't find anywhere else—comfort, control, belonging, escape?

_____

_____

_____

How has numbing betrayed you?

Name the ways it backfired—relational damage, health, shame, denial.

_____

_____

_____

What lies did you tell yourself to keep numbing—"It's not that bad," "Everyone does it," "I need this to cope"?

_____

_____

_____

What was your relationship with food growing up?

Was it comfort, control, punishment, reward?

_____

_____

_____

Did you ever use food to disappear—restricting so you wouldn't be noticed—or to fill emptiness, eating until the ache dulled?

What other numbing patterns have you used—work, sex, shopping, busyness, scrolling?

Write how they gave you relief and how they backfired.

What part of yourself is still waiting underneath the numbness, if you stopped dulling the pain long enough to listen?

Now Step Back and Look

Numbing is not the same as healing. It feels like control, but it steals it from you. It promises relief, but it robs you twice—once in the silence, and again when the pain returns heavier than before.

You are not weak for needing to escape. You were surviving. But survival cannot be the end of your story. There is more than spinning in the cycle of pain and relief, shame and silence. There is the slow, steady courage of facing the wound itself instead of covering it.

Drugs, alcohol, food, work, sex, shopping, distraction—they were never the problem. They were the strategy. They were the armor. They were the numbing agents you reached for because you were carrying what no child, no adult, no human being should ever have had to carry alone. That's not shameful. That's survival.

But now you have another choice. You can put the bottle down. You can step away from the binge or the fast. You can close the laptop, walk away from the purchase, put down the phone. You can refuse the lie that healing is too hard or too late. You can walk toward truth instead of hiding from it.

The drink, the pill, the plate, the rush, the noise—they don't own you. They don't define you. They don't get the last word. Healing does.

And boy did I learn how to numb. I learned from an early age to numb by doing creative arts and playing by myself in a corner. I learned had to shut down my emotions and only display to the world what was acceptable and pleasing to others. Year over year I learned that whoever I was was not acceptable. Not enough. I numbed through social alcohol addiction, weed smoking, exercise, shopping, lustful abandon with strangers, over performing at work, finding pride in all of my big paychecks, and hiding in a beautiful home surrounded by the facade of lies.

I learned that running and numbing almost cost me my life. I learned that I could not run from my own pain. I had to drop into the ashes and discover who I was free of numbing comforts. I had learned dissociating for hours was calming. Being lost in my own thoughts for days was offering protection from the world. I learned to isolate to continue my numbing behaviors. Left unchecked this practice nearly destroyed me.

Here's the truth. We need others in our life to support our efforts. We need trusted individuals that can help us see what we can't see on our own. Sometimes this is with a therapist, a trusted faith leader or a solid influence in our lives.

Breaking any cycle of numbing behaviors is hard. Let's face it – any change is hard. But the truth is you can not heal without a sober mind and a willing Spirit. If you start any new patterns because of this workbook hear this. You staying numb is exactly where the world wants to keep you. Wake up and step forward into freedom.

16

PAIN IS A MOTHERF#CKER

CHRONIC PAIN & ILLNESS AS THE BODY'S BURDEN

Pain doesn't care about your schedule, your deadlines, or your dreams. It barges in and takes up space in your body like it owns the place. Chronic pain is its own kind of abuser—demanding attention, stealing sleep, changing your plans, and reshaping your identity whether you want it to or not.

Pain doesn't just live in the body. It moves into your mind, your emotions, your sense of self. It whispers lies: "You're weak. You're broken. You'll never get better. You're a burden." And when it stays long enough, it starts to sound convincing.

Trauma makes this worse. Trauma trains your nervous system to live on high alert. Your brain becomes a smoke alarm stuck in overdrive. Pain rides that same pathway—every ache gets amplified, every flare feels like fire. The longer trauma and pain live together, the more they feed each other. The brain remembers the wound and keeps sounding the alarm even when the danger has passed. Trauma fuels the pain; pain fuels the trauma. It's a cycle that doesn't let up.

And then comes the isolation. Pain shrinks your world. Friends stop inviting you. Employers stop trusting you. Family stops believing you. Doctors dismiss you when your pain doesn't fit neatly into a test result. The loneliness of pain can feel heavier than the pain itself. Because pain doesn't just hurt your body—it rewrites your life until you hardly recognize it.

But here's the truth: pain may have invaded your body, but it doesn't define your worth. Illness is not weakness. Pain is not punishment. And struggling doesn't mean you've failed—it means you're human, carrying a body in a world that doesn't always know how to care for it.

Ask Yourself

What's the loudest lie pain tells you about your body or your worth? Write it down.

Is it saying you're weak? Broken? A burden? That you'll never get better? Sit with the first word that comes to mind — don't filter it.

_____

_____

_____

When you think about your pain, do you blame yourself?

Where did that belief start? Did someone teach you this? A parent? A doctor? A boss? Was it spoken directly, or did you just absorb it in silence? Trace the root.

_____

_____

_____

What labels have you heard from others (lazy, unreliable, weak) that made your pain heavier?

Whose voice do you still hear saying those words? How do those labels replay in your head today?

_____

_____

_____

What do you do to feed your own pain?

Is it pushing through when you need rest? Ignoring symptoms? Using food, substances, or overwork to cope? Be brutally honest about how you keep the cycle alive.

_____

_____

_____

Facing the Silence of Others—How has your family, workplace, or community minimized your pain?

Write their words.

_____

_____

_____

Was it "It's not that bad"? "Everyone hurts"? "You just need to toughen up"?

Capture the exact phrases — even if they sting.

_____

_____

_____

Who dismissed your illness because it "doesn't show"?

How did that land inside you? Did it make you doubt yourself? Did it make you angry? Did it make you quieter about what you were going through?

_____

_____

_____

What relationship or opportunity did pain cost you because someone couldn't handle your reality?

Was it a job? A marriage? A friendship? What did you lose because someone else chose denial over compassion?

_____

_____

_____

Now Step Back and Look

Reclaiming Your Truth

If your body could speak without shame, what would it say about what it has endured? Would it say "I'm tired"? "I've carried too much"? "I've survived hell and I'm still standing"? Let your body speak unfiltered.

What would it look like to stop apologizing for your pain?

Would it mean saying "no" without explaining? Resting without guilt? Speaking up when people dismiss you? Picture what unapologetic living looks like for you.

Finish this sentence: "Pain doesn't get to define me; I am _____."

You are not crazy for how much it hurts. Trauma wired your brain to sound alarms that don't shut off, and pain rides those signals like gasoline on fire. But that doesn't make you weak—it makes you human. You're not imagining it. You're not exaggerating it. Your body is telling the truth about what it's been through.

Pain isolates, but it doesn't erase you. Even if the world forgets you, dismisses you, or walks away, your presence still matters. Pain is loud, but it's not the whole story. You are still here. You are still breathing. And that matters more than what anyone else sees or believes.

Pain is a motherf#cker, but it's not your master. Go kick its ass every single day!

I live in chronic pain every single day. Most mornings it

feels like I'm rising out of a coffin just to get out of bed, and most nights it feels like I sink six inches into the mattress the moment I lie down. A decade ago I was diagnosed with severe fibromyalgia.

Fibromyalgia is one of the most misunderstood chronic illnesses out there. It isn't just "aches" or being tired. It's a full-body nervous system disorder where the pain signals never turn off. It's characterized by widespread musculoskeletal pain, deep fatigue, restless sleep, brain fog, and heightened sensitivity to even the smallest touch or noise. Doctors describe it as your pain volume being cranked all the way up — every signal amplified, every flare spreading like wildfire. What should feel like a light brush can feel like sandpaper or fire across your skin. What should be ordinary soreness becomes a body-wide alarm that never quiets.

Fibromyalgia is often linked with trauma — domestic abuse, childhood neglect, or repeated emotional injury. Trauma wires the brain to stay on high alert, and fibro hijacks that system. The nervous system is stuck in overdrive, firing signals that flood the body with pain. Trauma fuels the pain. Pain fuels the trauma. And the cycle doesn't stop.

Living with fibromyalgia feels like being trapped in the deep end of a pool. You can't swim up and you can't swim down — the pain just surrounds you, weighs you down, and doesn't let you breathe.

And yet people who don't live in it can't understand why you don't just buck up, take a couple Tylenol, or exercise more because "you'll feel better." They see a body that "looks fine" and assume you're exaggerating, lazy, or making excuses. But fibro is invisible — and invisibility is its own cruelty. It isolates you from belief, compassion, and empathy.

It's not my desire that everyone knows this pain. But it is my desire that people learn empathy for the pain they cannot see or understand. Because until empathy shows up, pain gets heavier — not lighter.

17

THE GILDED CAGE HAD GOLD LOCKS

SUCCESS THAT SUFFOCATES, AND WHAT FREEDOM ACTUALLY COSTS

*I*t looked like success — the salary, the title, the corner office, the perfectly curated version of your life. For a while, maybe it worked; you believed you had arrived. But here's what no one tells you about the top: it can be just as lonely, just as toxic, just as soul-suffocating as where you started. It just has better lighting.

This is the trap of the gilded cage. On the outside, it shines; inside, you're shrinking, bending, over-functioning, smiling while suffocating. You're succeeding — but it's costing you everything that matters. And the worst part? You're praised for it. They call you powerful, resilient, a go-getter. They don't see the pressure. They don't see what you've compromised just to be allowed in the room. This chapter is about what it costs to keep performing — and what it takes to finally walk away.

WHAT THE GILDED CAGE SOUNDS LIKE:

"I should be grateful."
"If I quit, they'll think I couldn't handle it."
"No one else here looks like me — I can't afford to fail."
"This job is killing me, but leaving feels like losing."
"I've worked too hard to throw it away."
"This is all I have left."

But when you zoom out, what you're really saying is: "I've chained myself to a version of success that no longer fits who I am." The longer you stay, the quieter your soul becomes.

~

Ask Yourself

What did "success" look like for you—and who sold you that vision?

Was it about money, image, approval, survival, or all of the above? What did you sacrifice to get there?

_____

_____

_____

What part of you knew, even in your best moments, that something wasn't right?

Did you feel disconnected? Misaligned? Exhausted? What signs did you ignore?

_____

_____

_____

Who benefited from your ability to hold it all together?

Who got comfort, power, or prestige while you were silently crumbling?

_____

_____

_____

What golden handcuffs kept you tied to the cage?

Financial security? Reputation? Fear of starting over? Fear of being forgotten?

_____

_____

_____

When did the version of success you were chasing start to feel like a prison?

Was it a moment, a season, a series of compromises? Name what turned.

_____

_____

_____

If you could rebuild your life around peace—not performance— what would it actually look like?

Write it down. No titles. No accolades. Just alignment.

_____

_____

_____

Now Step Back and Look

You didn't sell out. You survived. You built something from nothing. You climbed. You conquered. You adapted. But now you're allowed to admit the truth: the cage was gilded — but it was still a cage. You weren't free. You were tolerated. You were rewarded for compliance, not truth. You played the game so well they forgot you were a human being. Maybe you forgot too.

Now you see it. Here's the question: will you stay for the image, or will you leave for the life you were actually meant to live? Freedom costs. It will cost you reputation, comfort, applause. But it will give you back your voice, your rest, your soul. You are not weak for leaving what looked like everything. You are wise for finally choosing what was real.

Writing about my years in corporate and the abuse leveled at me in those hallowed walls was harder than exploring where my childhood and young-adult trauma actually began. I realized that daily I was still stuck in the same cage of expectations that had been placed on me as a young girl — unrealistic expectations to look the other way, go along with the crowd, never bring anything wrong to anyone's attention, and never speak up. I got angry.

Once inside a system where few people get to actually thrive, I had been completely minimized. These weren't accidental wounds — these were strategic cuts to my underbelly: direct shaming and guilt applied with precision. But the difference here was that the system provided my financial security, my safety, and my identity. It was a conundrum for sure.

Just like in childhood, I was reminded that I should be grateful and that I should show thankfulness at every offense — and never raise my voice to defend myself. I realized something else: no one at the corporate tables where I sat looked like me. I was female. I was a token of their choosing, all too happy to have a seat at the table.

When I looked back at all the stories, all the mocking, all the minimization, and all the corporate grooming, I realized I had proof: proof that an honest person can survive at these tables; proof that a paycheck doesn't mean you have to bow to twisted ethics and corporate games; proof that I couldn't play dumb just to make others comfortable. I'd tried that in high school — it didn't work — and it certainly did not work in corporate America.

So I started speaking. I started telling the truth, unashamedly. And I was shut down, closed out, shown the door — every time. Even after being physically assaulted by a co-worker, I was told I was only 50% of the problem. But it was me who had to go.

18

I WAS THE SECRET THEY COULDN'T CONTROL

OWNING YOUR VOICE AFTER BEING SILENCED, SHAMED, OR EXILED

They never expected you to speak. They expected you to comply. To stay small. To keep their secrets. To carry the shame they created—and stay quiet about the truth you lived. Because your silence served them. Your obedience made them feel safe. Your disappearance protected their image.

But then you started remembering. Then you started naming. Then you started talking—and the whole narrative began to unravel. This chapter is about that unraveling. The moment you realized you weren't the problem. You were the proof. Proof of what they did. Proof of what they denied. Proof of the truth they buried. And that made you dangerous.

Why They Tried to Silence You:

• *Because your honesty threatened their control*

• *Because your healing exposed their dysfunction*

• *Because your strength made their manipulation look weak*

• *Because your memory was too vivid to rewrite*

• Because your presence proved the damage was real

You weren't too loud.

You weren't unstable.

You weren't imagining it.

You were simply no longer *controllable.*

Ask Yourself

Who made you feel unsafe for telling the truth?

What did they say? What did they deny? What did they rewrite to protect themselves?

When were you exiled, discarded, or ghosted for speaking up?

Who turned their back when you needed them to stand with you? What lie did they tell to justify it?

What secrets did you hold that were never yours to carry?

Abuse? Infidelity? Addiction? Dysfunction? Who benefited from your silence?

What did it cost you to stay quiet?

Emotionally, physically, spiritually—how did that silence affect your identity?

_____

_____

_____

What part of your voice still feels shaky today?

What truths still feel dangerous to say out loud?

_____

_____

_____

What would it look like to tell your story without apology or permission?

Where would you begin? Who would you stop trying to protect? What would finally be free?

_____

_____

_____

Now Step Back and Look

You were never the problem. You were the inconvenient truth. They didn't silence you because you were wrong. They silenced you because you were right—and unstoppable if anyone listened.

But here's what they never counted on: that you'd find your voice anyway, that you'd live to tell it, that you'd no longer shrink in their shadow. You don't owe anyone a sanitized version of what you lived through. You don't have to apologize for surviving it—and naming it. The ones who tried to shame you never had your best interest in mind. They had their own reputations in mind. Their own comfort. Their own power.

But your life is not a PR campaign. And your voice is not on loan. You are the proof they can't erase. You are the truth they couldn't contain. You are the secret they couldn't control—because now you're speaking. And this time, you're not asking for permission.

> *Looking over all the chapters of my book that I have written—the ones still needing editing, still demanding my full attention—I realized one thing: I was a secret they couldn't control. I was the one who spoke too loudly. The one who told the truth in rooms built on lies. The one they never knew what would come out of my mouth—and were secretly afraid of.*
>
> *I had a story to tell. A story about a life of abuse—and the many ways I fed into my own abusive thoughts, actions,*

and reactions. It was hard to determine which secrets I would share, which ones I would carry quietly in my heart and soul, and which ones I would never go back to again.

But once I began to understand what complex trauma really does—how it distorts perception, how it sabotages connection, how it rewires your ability to relate to others—I felt a wave of relief. I'm not ashamed of my past. I'm not ashamed of the person I used to be. And I am certainly not ashamed of the woman I am today.

I wasn't afraid to put the stories of shame out into the world—both the shame that was imposed on me and the shame I carried inside myself. Because I'm done with secrets. Secrets destroyed my soul. They stole my health. They hijacked my ability to navigate this world in the name of being liked, accepted, and valued. They had to be revealed. And they had to be released.

I now know—I was never the problem. I was just the inconvenient truth-teller. A woman who held herself down in her own darkness for too long so others wouldn't feel exposed by her light

19

LOVE DOESN'T GHOST YOU

NAMING ABANDONMENT, ESTRANGEMENT, AND WHAT REAL LOVE REQUIRES

*T*hey didn't die. They just stopped calling. They just stopped showing up. They just slowly erased you—until one day, it was clear: you were no longer in their life. No fight. No closure. No explanation. Just distance dressed up as "boundaries," just silence wearing the mask of "peace."

But let's be honest: love doesn't ghost you. Fear does. Shame does. Control does. But love—real love—shows up. Even when it's hard. Especially when it's hard. This chapter is for the ones left behind: the mothers unfriended by their sons, the daughters blamed for breaking cycles they didn't choose, the partners abandoned after the mask slipped, the friends ghosted the moment they got honest. This is where we stop blaming ourselves for someone else's retreat—and start defining love by truth, not trauma.

WHAT ESTRANGEMENT FEELS LIKE:

- Invisible grief with no funeral.
- Being punished for healing.
- Having to explain what they won't admit.
- Feeling erased while they rewrite the narrative.
- Loving someone who acts like you never existed.

It's not just sad. It's disorienting. You ask yourself: Was any of it real? Did I do something unforgivable? Will they ever come back? But here's the answer your healing needs most: their silence is not your shame to carry.

∾

ASK YOURSELF

Who ghosted you—and what did they leave behind?

Write their name. Name the hole. What story did they never let you finish?

_____

_____

_____

How did they justify their absence?

"It's better this way"? "You're toxic"? "I need space"? What truth did they dodge?

_____

_____

_____

What have you blamed yourself for that was actually their unwillingness to engage?

Did you over-apologize? Did you keep reaching out? What did you try to fix that wasn't yours?

_____

_____

_____

What memories still haunt you because there was no closure?

What would you say if they gave you five minutes of honesty?

_____

_____

_____

Have you confused silence with peace?

What's the emotional toll of pretending you're unbothered?

_____

_____

_____

What would it look like to let go—not with hate, but with clarity?

What would you release? What would you stop expecting?

_____

_____

_____

NOW STEP BACK AND LOOK

People will ghost you and call it growth. They'll disappear and say they were protecting their peace. They'll remove you from their life and claim it was healing. But healing doesn't punish. Love doesn't exile. And boundaries without communication are not boundaries—they're brick walls.

You've been carrying a grief no one talks about: the grief of being unwanted while still alive; the grief of being erased without explanation; the grief of knowing the person you love is alive and well—just not in your life. So here's the truth: if someone can leave without a word, they were never capable of the love you were giving. If someone makes you beg for access, it was never intimacy—it was control. If someone ghosts you when you start speaking truth, they were never listening to begin with. Let them go. Let them rewrite. Let them forget.

But you? You remember who you are. You name what happened. You grieve what was real. And then you rise—not bitter, but clear. Because love doesn't ghost you. It shows up. It listens. It stays—even when it's hard.

I had to take a hard look at my emotional support network—family, friends, coworkers, and those calling them- selves Christians. When I considered the deep, unshakable love I have for my Father, I knew what real love felt like. So I turned that same mirror—that microscope—back onto my relationships. And the truth showed up fast.

I had poured into people who only took. I helped, I gave, I carried them—financially, emotionally, spiritually. But once Christ revealed the trauma I'd been living in, I saw how I had played possum in relationships for years—never asking for anything in return. It's painful, knowing the list of those who've turned away. I know every name. I know when the kindness stopped. I know when the phone stopped ringing. And I realized—I had been left behind by every person I thought loved me.

But you know what? Relief. Freedom. Never going back. In my workbook, I asked: What would it look like to let go—not with hate, but with clarity? This is what it looks like. And it feels like peace.

Love is of Christ. Worldly love is fleeting—shallow, predictable. Christ loves you in brokenness and wholeness—His love never leaves. His love doesn't ghost. It stays. It grows. It walks with you through every season. If you don't know that kind of love—I'm sorry. I didn't either. Until I did.

20

THE DISGUISES OF WOUNDED HUNGER—GREED, MONEY, AND IDOLS

NAMING WHAT SUCCESS IS HIDING—SO PROTECTION CAN BECOME HEALING, NOT ANOTHER PRISON.

Greed rarely starts as greed. It begins as ache: the hollow stomach of neglect, the empty home where love was absent, the small child who learned that achievement got applause while pain got ignored. Success becomes armor. Money becomes anesthesia. You don't call it idolatry—you call it survival. But the truth is, greed and idols cover what trauma carved: a need for control after chaos, a hunger for approval after rejection, a grasp for safety after being left unprotected.

When you've been unseen, achievement becomes your spotlight. When you've been powerless, money becomes your sword. When you've been discarded, success becomes your proof you should have been chosen. And for a while, it works: the job titles drown out the voices of shame; the possessions dress the wounds in something shiny; the ladder climbing feels like rising above it all. But underneath—the ache remains. Because trauma doesn't dissolve in paychecks. It waits, whispering at night after the applause dies down, asking if you're really safe now, if you're really loved, if you're really enough.

GREED AND IDOLS IN TRAUMA OFTEN LOOK LIKE:

- perfectionism that hides the child who was told they'd never measure up;
- overwork that numbs the body's memory of powerlessness;
- status symbols that silence the shame of being unseen;
- buying love because real intimacy feels unsafe;
- achievement addiction that masks fear of abandonment;
- envy that is really grief—longing for what others got freely and you never did;
- control that keeps the nervous system from collapsing under chaos.

This isn't drama—it's survival disguised as ambition. And you are allowed to grieve the false idols you built your life upon, only to discover they were scaffolding over pain. The job that stamped you with worth but never knew your name. The house you stuffed with things so it wouldn't echo with emptiness. The applause that muted shame but never healed it. The image of strength that was really a terrified child in costume. You don't owe anyone a polished story about why you chased success. Sometimes survival looked like greed. Sometimes striving was camouflage. But here's the truth—idols don't just dissolve, they have to be smashed. And you hold the hammer.

Every time you name what was false, you swing. Every time you refuse to sacrifice yourself for applause, you swing. Every time you choose presence over performance, you swing. The altar begins to crack. The mask begins to fall. And when it shatters, you are left with what is real: the ache, the hunger, the child who needed love more than accolades.

That child deserves more than scaffolding. That child deserves truth. And smashing idols is how you finally give it. The endless pursuit of money will not provide security , love, self-confidence or peace, but it can sure rob us of it.

∾

Ask Yourself

What wound was covered by your pursuit of money or success?

Name it plainly—abandonment, fear, shame, loneliness, invisibility.

What did achievement give you that childhood did not?

Write the difference between applause and nurture, between recognition and love.

When did "more" feel like safety?

Trace the first memory where earning, winning, or buying felt like protection.

What cost have you paid to keep the image intact?

Health, sleep, relationships, faith—name what was sacrificed on the altar.

_____

_____

_____

What is your body telling you when the striving stops?

Notice the anxiety, the emptiness, the trembling beneath the silence.

_____

_____

_____

If you could bless the child who thought success would finally make them safe, what would you say?

Write it. Speak it aloud. Let it land as truth.

_____

_____

_____

What practice will allow you to feel worth without earning it?

Stillness, prayer, therapy, play, honesty—choose one and name it.

_____

_____

_____

NOW STEP BACK AND LOOK

Success is not evil. Money is not shameful. Greed is not always born from arrogance. Sometimes it is born from wounds. Trauma teaches the lie that worth must be earned, that safety must be bought, that love must be proven. And greed, money, and idols become the cover story— the armor, the mask, the distraction.

You are not wrong for building armor when you were unprotected. You are not shallow for chasing applause when you were ignored. You are not weak for numbing hunger with "more." You were surviving. But survival is not the same as healing.

Now you can choose different. You can let provision be a gift, not idols. You can let success be fruit, not identity. You can let money serve you instead of mastering you. You can listen to the child underneath the striving and finally say: You are already enough. You are already safe. You are already loved.

This is not losing. This is laying down the mask. And in the laying down, you don't shrink—you become whole.

> I lived 20+ years of my life in corporate America wanting more and more and more. I found respect, accolades, and financial success—but the emptiness remained. Sure, greed was driving me, but it was also lust, validation, desperation, and an envy of myself that had no bounds.
>
> I built my world like an elaborate castle: my home, my cars, my vacations, my happy-looking family, my pretty

friends, my great career, my extensive traveling—all topped off with quarterly bonuses. It was endless. I used the world as my playground.

Until I couldn't go any faster. I couldn't spread myself any thinner. I couldn't turn off the machine I had become. Like a robot. A walking billboard of emptiness.

Greed had become unquenchable. But honestly, the money was just a by-product. What I was really searching for was acceptance. Inclusion. Such a simple thing to want— yet for me it was always out of reach.

21

BREAKING THE SILENCE

FAITH, MENTAL HEALTH, AND ACCEPTANCE

From church pews to boardrooms to barracks — ending the shame of mental illness.

Silence has long been the weapon of choice when it comes to mental illness. It does not shout, it strangles. It does not heal, it hides. It does not protect, it poisons. In families, silence protects an image while children suffocate under the weight of unspoken pain. In churches, it dresses itself in piety with phrases like "just pray harder" while people quietly bleed in the pews. In the workplace, silence wears the mask of professionalism, recasting breakdowns as mere stress and punishing anyone who admits they cannot keep up. In the military, silence masquerades as strength, forcing wounded soldiers to fight wars inside their own minds with no brotherhood beside them.

Silence is efficient. It keeps systems polished, reputations intact, and uncomfortable truths buried. But it is never neutral. Silence is a verdict, a declaration that your pain is too much, your struggle is unwelcome, your voice is dangerous, and your existence is inconvenient. The cost is staggering. Generations of Christians mistake depression for a lack of faith. Soldiers return from combat alive only to die quietly by their own hand. Professionals climb corporate ladders while collapsing in secret. Families gather around dinner tables with smiles plastered on their faces while every person in the room knows exactly what cannot be spoken.

Silence doesn't just ignore mental illness; it feeds it. Shame grows in the dark. Isolation deepens the wound. And the longer silence rules, the harder it becomes to speak at all. But here is the truth that must be named: silence is not holy, judgment is not healing, and shame is not of Christ.

IN THE CHURCH

When mental illness is mentioned in the church, it is often met with suspicion or pity. Depression is dismissed as a lack of faith. Suicidal thoughts are judged as demonic and is prayed for. Anxiety is reframed as prayerlessness. PTSD and childhood trauma is treated like rebellion to Gods sovereignty to heal all things. Bipolar disorder is quietly avoided because no one knows what to do with it. The tragedy is that the very place meant to be a hospital for the broken often becomes the most unsafe place to bleed. People sit through sermons carrying panic, despair, or flashbacks, but dare not speak for fear of being labeled as spiritually defective. Instead of finding refuge, they learn that disclosure comes at the cost of credibility. They pray harder, not because they believe healing depends on it, but because they know their pain must be disguised as devotion.

~

Ask Yourself

When someone says "mental illness," what is the first judgment that rises in your heart—faithless, unstable, dangerous?

Write it down.

_____

_____

_____

When did you use prayer as a substitute for professional help?

What happened afterward?

If a member who has a metal disorder admitted suicidal ideation, would you embrace them—acting like they are broken vessels, with all the sad faces and self-righteous superiority you can't hide or quietly slide away and gossip?

Have you ever been more concerned with preserving the church's image than protecting someone's life?

Be honest.

IN THE FAMILY

In families, silence wears a different mask. It shows up in phrases like, "We don't talk about that," "Just get over it," or "You're too sensitive." Parents keep and impose secrets to protect reputations. Siblings collude in silence to keep the myth of a perfect home alive. Children learn early that performance is the price of belonging, while pain is an inconvenience best hidden in bedrooms and journals. Generations pass along this inheritance of suppression, teaching each child to silence their voice before anyone else can. It's called generational trauma and it is abuse. Behind closed doors, everyone knows who struggles with addiction, depression, or eating disorders, but the rules are clear: the story cannot be spoken. The family image must remain intact, even if every member inside it is breaking.

~

What phrase did your family use to shut you down—"stop crying," "toughen up," "don't embarrass us," "It wasnt that bad"?

Write the exact words.

_____

_____

_____

Who in your family carried a hidden struggle everyone saw but no one dared name?

Write their name.

How much silence did you inherit to keep the family myth intact?

"Don't tell. Don't ask."

What truth about your family would shatter the image if it were spoken aloud?

IN THE WORKPLACE

The workplace is no different. Mental illness is recast into labels that strip people of dignity. Depression is mistaken for laziness. Anxiety is brushed off as dramatics. PTSD is coded as instability. People hide therapy appointments, medication, and even hospitalizations because they know disclosure could stall promotions or mark them as unfit. Workplaces claim to value well-being, but most reward overwork while quietly punishing anyone who admits they are struggling. Leaders will praise productivity while ignoring the toll it takes on body and mind. The result is a culture where silence feels safer than honesty, even as the cost of silence mounts in burnout, breakdown, and resignation.

$\sim$

Which mental illnesses are most mislabeled where you work?

Depression called "lazy"? Anxiety called "dramatic"? PTSD called "unstable"? Write them out.

_____

_____

_____

Have you hidden therapy, medication, or hospitalization from your boss?

What were you afraid they would say?

_____

_____

_____

Does your company hand out wellness slogans while rewarding burnout?

Write the contradiction.

What unwritten rule in your workplace says that silence is safer than honesty?

IN THE MILITARY

In the military, silence is baptized as strength. Soldiers learn quickly that wounds you can see are honored with medals, but wounds you cannot see are branded as weakness. PTSD is spoken of in whispers, if at all. Depression is met with suspicion. Suicidal thoughts are buried under bravado, because admitting them risks your standing, your reputation, even your brothers' respect. Those who do speak risk being labeled, sidelined, or discharged. Silence becomes the currency of survival. But the price is devastating. Service members who returned alive from war lose their lives at home in a quieter, lonelier battle. Entire platoons carry unspoken scars, while the culture insists that strength means silence, even as silence steals lives.

～

What is the unspoken message about PTSD—cowardice, instability, weakness?

Write the truth, not the slogan.

_____

_____

_____

What happens to soldiers who admit mental health struggles—do they get help, or do they get marked?

_____

_____

_____

How has silence about suicide cost lives in your unit, your barracks, your community?

Write the number that still haunts you.

_____

_____

_____

When did you learn that silence equals survival, and how much has it cost you?

A marriage? A relationship? Job? Peace?

Now Step Back and Look

Not every wound bleeds where others can see it. Mental illness often hides in plain sight, masked by smiles, success, or silence. And when the pain is not visible, the world insists it is not real. That lie keeps millions fighting battles the Church, family, workplace, and military refuse to name. Depression hides behind polite smiles and repeated claims of "I'm fine." Anxiety hides behind over-preparing, over-performing, and people-pleasing. Obsessive-Compulsive Disorder hides behind rituals dismissed as quirks or perfectionism. Bipolar disorder hides behind bursts of energy praised as ambition, and crashes endured in silence. PTSD hides behind hypervigilance, avoidance, nightmares, and panic when memories return. Complex PTSD hides behind dissociation, trust issues, relational chaos, and shame born from repeated trauma. Eating disorders hide behind restriction praised as discipline, or overeating drowned in guilt and secrecy. Addiction hides behind medals, ministry, work ethic, and overachievement.

But here is the truth: if it does not show, it is still real. Hidden does not mean fake. Unseen does not mean weak. And silence has never healed anyone.

You are not wrong for struggling. You are not faithless for needing help. You are not weak for telling the truth. Breaking the silence is not rebellion. It is redemption. Because when the Church, the family, the workplace, and the military stop demanding silence, the wounded stop dying in it. And the truth finally gets the last word.

I was sixty years old when I received my diagnosis of

complex childhood trauma—C-PTSD. For the first time, I began to understand the abusive cycles I had been living in and the old patterns I thought I had overcome, patterns that were really driven by trauma coping strategies. I wasn't living. I was just surviving.

For thirty years I moved at the speed of light in my career, going everywhere but nowhere fast. Eventually, I collapsed. The pain had to stop. I checked myself into Sabino Trauma Treatment Center and began to heal. It was freeing to dig into my secrets with world-class therapists and to learn tools such as Eye Movement Desensitization and Reprocessing (EMDR), Accelerated Resolution Therapy (ART), biofeedback, and brain work. For the first time, I could see clearly where my mental illness had originated.

The root was simple and devastating: the day I was rejected by my mother—at birth.

That knowledge was life-changing. I released the shame of her rejection and finally accepted that I had been conditioned to take abuse in childhood, marriages, in motherhood, in corporate politics, and in deeply ingrained friendships.

But everything changed when I put all of the shame down. When I said, "No more." When I quit playing the game so many had counted on me continuing. I stood up and started living the life I had owned from the day I was born but had been denied. Now I live free, at peace, and protected.

Not everyone was happy that I began unashamedly telling those in my circle about my awakening to complex trauma and the clarity it brought to my life. They wanted everything to go back to how it was before. They didn't like the "new Jo." And I understand why. The old Jo could be used. The old Jo could be manipulated by guilt or shame, her emotions twisted to keep her pliable. That version of me didn't set boundaries or hold them.

The old Jo tolerated gaslighting at work, disguised as "new direction." She minimized sexism as a nuisance. She groused at corporate culture disguised as intimidation, the kind that weaponized hierarchy, rewarded silence, and called abuse "leadership." She had lived long enough inside board-rooms where gaslighting was rebranded as strategy, exclusion was labeled efficiency, and bullying was dressed up as accountability. She knew what it was: intimidation, plain and simple, a system built to shrink the voices of anyone who dared to resist. Sure she complained when she was shut out of meetings or reduced to a token voice at the table, - But the new Jo?! She could not be silenced. The new Jo reported when a male coworker physically attacked her, only to discover that HR dismissed her because she had admitted to disassociating. "She actually hosted a call with teammates and leaders to discuss her mental illness- "Didn't you hear?"

The old Jo was shamed in church for the strength of her testimony of Christ and told to tone it down to keep others comfortable. And she stayed anyway. But the new Jo wrote a book about her mental health struggles, exposing shame and pointing to Christ as the source of her peace and stability.

All the voices of others about your shortcomings were not meant to build you up, but tear you down. Drown out the negative voices and live free.

For me, - My mother's words—"You rejected me as a baby. If abortion had been legal, you wouldn't be here"— finally lost their sting. I'm here- and I'm not going anywhere.

Today, I get to be just me. When you dare to dig into the darkest corners of your story and lay the truth out for the *world to see, shame loses its power. You realize you have nothing to lose and everything to gain.*

PART III

Reclaiming Truth

This Stage is about taking back what survival and breaking tried to steal. Not pretending you're fine. Not skipping over scars. Reclaiming truth means standing in it — that you didn't cause this, that you're not defined by pain, that healing is messy but possible. Here, you don't just survive. You don't just break. You rise with truth in your hands, ready to call yourself whole even if the world doesn't understand it.

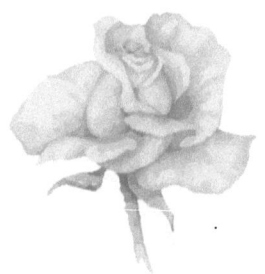

22

YOU DIDN'T CAUSE THIS, YOU'RE JUST CARRYING IT

COMING TO GRIPS WITH YOURSELF

*Y*ou didn't ask for this. You didn't sit down and choose panic attacks, flashbacks, emotional shutdown, or the fear of getting close. You didn't want the hyper-vigilance, the shame spiral, the need to control everything just to feel safe. But here you are—carrying it all. Still showing up. Still breathing. Still fighting to explain the invisible war inside you that most people don't even believe exists. This chapter is about that war, about the damage that didn't start with you but lives inside you now, about the difference between fault and responsibility. You didn't cause this. You're just carrying it. And now? You're allowed to put some of it down.

What Complex PTSD feels like, even when you don't know it yet, can include feeling unsafe even in safe spaces, always waiting for the other shoe to drop, numbness you can't explain followed by waves of rage or grief, deep shame without a clear reason, being overly responsible for others or completely detached, exhaustion that sleep can't fix, emotional flashbacks that feel like overreactions to "normal" moments, and isolation even around people you love. This isn't weakness; this is your nervous system still trying to protect you from a past that isn't over yet.

～

Ask Yourself

When did you first start thinking something was "wrong" with you?

What symptoms did you notice? Who ignored, mocked, or misdiagnosed them?

_____

_____

_____

What messages did you receive about mental illness growing up?

Were you taught to hide it, pray it away, push through it, or fear it? How did those beliefs affect your healing?

_____

_____

_____

Who made you believe your pain was your fault?

What did they say? What did they accuse you of? How did they twist your trauma into a personal failure?

_____

_____

_____

What are the survival patterns you once relied on—but now feel heavy to carry?

Perfectionism? Avoidance? Rage? Silence? Write what you're still holding that doesn't feel like *you*.

_____

_____

_____

What part of your story are you still punishing yourself for, even though it wasn't your fault?

Say it clearly. Say it without defending anyone else.

_____

_____

_____

What would healing look like if it wasn't about fixing yourself—but about understanding yourself?

How would you treat your symptoms differently? How would you speak to your mind, your body, your past?

_____

_____

_____

Now Step Back and Look

Mental illness is not a character flaw. Complex PTSD is not a death sentence. And you? You're not broken—you're burdened, burdened by pain that was never meant to be yours in the first place. You adapted. You survived. You took on the weight that others refused to acknowledge. You internalized chaos so others could maintain appearances. You blamed yourself because no one else wanted to be accountable. But it's time to say what no one else did: it wasn't your fault—not the way you froze, not the way you lashed out, not the way you clung, ran, or shut down. You didn't cause this. You're just carrying it. And now, you're allowed to understand it, to name it, to stop shaming yourself for how you've responded to things no one else had to survive.

You may have inherited trauma, but you don't have to pass it on. You may still be healing, but you don't have to stay hidden. This isn't about pretending you're okay; this is about telling the truth so you don't have to keep pretending at all. You didn't cause this. You're just carrying it. And now, finally—you get to choose what to carry forward.

So—crafting my book took a minute or two, until I realized life is a full circle, and that's exactly how I needed to lay out this book. It's not neat. It's not tidy. There is no bow at the end. There are twists, wrong starts, bad starts, faulty starts. But ultimately, everything we do in life brings us right back to the moment you're in right now—reading my words. Healing doesn't look like perfection. Healing isn't easy. Healing takes work, not just the kind you do in your own mind. You must reach for professional help. You must seek out community. You must cling to a tight circle of people who love you for real.

Healing is exercise. Just like growing your muscles, you have to do it every single day. You must get up every day and continue your healing path like your life depends on it—because it does. You need to understand clearly what triggers you, what sends you sideways, and what brings you peace. None of these steps can be left out. It needs to become as routine as brushing your teeth, brushing your hair, and taking a shower. Healing must be part of your daily life.

Let's face it: the fact that anyone actually wants you to heal—to be strong, to be vocal, to be opinionated, to say such vulnerable truth—is rare. Many people are very happy with how it's been all along. They don't want change. Especially not from someone they've gotten used to using for whatever they needed.

Boundary setting is hard. Boundary setting is lonely. Boundary setting is the only way you are ever going to step up, step out, and rise into your healing. If you can't take this basic step, I'm going to tell you something hard: your path back to peace, to contentment, to joy will be incredibly difficult or nonexistent.

Sorry, I'm not here to blow smoke up your ass. It's hard, continual work. But it's worth every step, every breath, every boundary. And if you've made it this far—you're already doing it.

23

THIS ISN'T A TESTIMONY — IT'S A TAKE-BACK

REWRITING YOUR NARRATIVE—NOT TO INSPIRE OTHERS, BUT TO FINALLY LIVE. TO HEAL

They'll say, "What a testimony." They'll say, "You've been through so much." They'll say, "God must be using your pain for something beautiful." And maybe He is. But this isn't about them. This isn't a highlight reel. This isn't a redemption arc curated for their comfort. This isn't you standing in your trauma for someone else's inspiration. This is a take-back. A taking back of power. Of your name. Of your truth. Of your full, unedited life. Because too many people have clapped for your healing without ever acknowledging your hell. Too many have tried to slap a "praise report" sticker on a story they never had to survive. Too many have used your survival to avoid their own reckoning. This chapter isn't for the ones watching. It's for you.

WHAT TAKING IT BACK SOUNDS LIKE:

"I don't need your applause to know I survived."
"I'm not here to inspire you—I'm here to live."
"This story belongs to me now."
"Healing isn't a performance."
"God didn't do this to me—but He did get me through it."

When you take your life back, you stop asking for validation. You stop shrinking your story to fit a testimony box. You stop letting others define what counts as healing.

~

Ask Yourself

What parts of your story have you edited to protect others' comfort?

What details have you downplayed? What truth have you coated in sugar so people wouldn't flinch?

_____

_____

_____

Who tried to use your survival to make themselves feel better?

Who told you "everything happens for a reason"? Who tried to fast-forward your grief?

_____

_____

_____

What version of you was praised for enduring pain—but never acknowledged for speaking truth?

Were you called strong—but not believed? Were you celebrated for "overcoming" what no one helped you through?

What would your story sound like if you stopped trying to make it inspiring—and just made it *honest*?

No edits. No bows. Just raw, real, unflinching truth. What's the version that sets *you* free?

What does taking your life back look like, practically?

What boundaries shift? What conversations end? What masks come off?

Where have you made survival your identity—and what would it feel like to just *live* again?

Not prove. Not to teach. Not to rise above. Just to *be*.

_____

_____

_____

Now Step Back and Look

This is not a performance. This is not a memoir for marketability. This is not the part where you hand the mic to someone else so they can "learn" from your pain. This is the part where you take your story back from every hand that tried to hold it without honoring it.

You are not a brand. You are not a symbol. You are not a quote on someone else's timeline. You are a person who lived. Who bled. Who crawled out of the wreckage. And you're still here. Not because of how the story sounds—but because of what it cost. So if this is a testimony, let it testify to this: they don't get to write the ending. You do. Take it back. All of it. And this time—keep it.

So when I wrapped up the final design of my book—with all the pictures of my life, and all the stories I chose to tell—I realized it was a reckoning, not just a testimony. I had cleared my past sins. I had pronounced all of the glory to Christ. And I was relieved by the rawness of my writing. I had bled out the trauma-filled shame and silence. I had offered hope between the pages—pages that held deplorable actions and deeds I had done in my past. It was so refreshing.

My testimony of Christ has always been an easy one to tell: I was once a deplorable sinner—but now, under His grace and undeserved mercy, I am His prize and His crown. I don't need others to reaffirm what I already know is true in my heart and soul. And that's the beauty of taking back your testimony.

24

HEALING LOOKS LIKE THIS

CHOOSING WHOLENESS OVER SURVIVAL— AGAIN AND AGAIN

*H*ealing doesn't look like perfection. It looks like choice. It looks like return. It looks like finally telling the truth and refusing to walk it back. It's not always graceful. It doesn't always look "healed." It looks like shaking hands while setting a boundary. It looks like saying, "I'm not okay," and not apologizing for it. It looks like walking out of the room you once begged to be let into. It looks like sobbing through a hard conversation—and still finishing it. Healing isn't a mountaintop moment. It's a slow, sacred rebellion, a refusal to live one more day as the version of you someone else shaped in fear.

Healing looks like knowing your triggers and showing up anyway. It looks like letting the phone ring and not feeling guilty. It looks like saying "no" without a novel of explanation. It looks like feeling grief and not needing to perform gratitude. It looks like hearing the inner critic and not letting it drive you. It looks like noticing your trauma response —and choosing a different one. It looks like crying without shame, laughing without apology, and resting without guilt.

~

ASK YOURSELF

What does healing *actually* look like for you right now—not what others expect it to be?

Messy? Quiet? Lonely? Fierce? Write the version that's *true*.

_____

_____

_____

What old roles, responses, or stories no longer fit who you're becoming?

What are you ready to release? Whose voice are you ready to stop obeying?

_____

_____

_____

What's something you've done recently that your old self would've never believed was possible?

Name it. Claim it. *That* is healing.

_____

_____

_____

What truth are you finally ready to live out loud?

Even if no one claps. Even if no one agrees. Even if it costs you comfort. Write it here.

What promise will you keep to yourself this time?

Not for them. Not to prove. Just for *you.*

Now Step Back and Look

You've faced the mirror. You've named the silence. You've grieved what didn't go right. You've told the truth no one else was willing to say. You've walked through trauma, betrayal, addiction, abandonment, and shame—and you're still standing. Not because you were rescued, but because you refused to disappear. Healing didn't find you. You found it. You dug it up with your bare hands. You pulled it out of grief, out of flashbacks, out of hospital beds and courtroom silence and corporate betrayal. You earned this wholeness. And now you know: it's not soft. It's not sweet. It's not for show. It's a fire. A rebuilding. A takeback. Healing means choosing not to live one more day as someone else's version of you. It means waking up every morning and saying, "I choose me. I choose truth. I choose peace—even if it costs everything I once called success." You've carried the wound. You've carried the shame. Now carry the freedom. This is healing. And it looks like you.

So—look at yourself. Really look. This is what I did when I finally took a hard look in the mirror. I had to clearly see all the trauma markers that had plagued me for the past sixty-two years and, if I'm honest, still continue to plague me. I came to grips with what I saw in the mirror, and I had to admit: my reflection was never who I really was. The mirror was never the enemy. What was living within me—thriving within my mind—that was the enemy.

I had to work hard to reclaim the semblance of peace I had created by beginning to heal. Of all my past actions, my past hurts, and my past hangups—I had to shed them in order to break free. I had to believe that I was never broken. Getting back to the woman I was before I started this path of healing was never the goal. Not even becoming the woman I am today. The goal? Becoming the woman I will be. The woman who moves forward every day knowing with full certainty that she will never return to her past.

That woman is me. That woman is you. And now? That woman is strong. She is confident. She walks in the truth that she was never the one to blame, and in the full understanding that none of this healing could've ever been done without Christ's orchestration.

25

ANGER ISN'T THE ENEMY—
DENIAL IS

REFRAMING ANGER AS A SIGNAL OF
INJUSTICE AND A TOOL FOR HEALING

*Y*ou weren't supposed to get mad. You were supposed to stay quiet, be understanding, be patient, be polite, and be small. You were taught that anger makes you dangerous, that it is the opposite of grace, and that it means you've lost control.

But here's the truth: your anger was never the problem. Their denial was. You weren't wrong to feel what you felt; you were just punished for noticing. Anger is not sin—it is a signal, a holy flare in the dark that says, something is not right here. In a world where trauma is minimized, injustice is dismissed, and survivors are told to "get over it," anger becomes sacred.

It's what wakes you up. It's what brings your voice back. It's what separates who you are from what you've endured. This chapter isn't about rage—it's about righteous clarity, the kind that says, I see what happened, and I'm not pretending anymore.

What Suppressed Anger Looks Like:

Smiling while seething. Chronic fatigue or illness. Explosive outbursts over small things. Guilt for setting boundaries. Discomfort with confrontation. Anxiety masked as people-pleasing. Freezing or shutting down during conflict.

When you've been told your anger is dangerous, you learn to stuff it deep—until it leaks out sideways. That's not healing; that's survival. And it doesn't have to stay that way.

~

ASK YOURSELF

What made you believe your anger wasn't allowed?

Who taught you it was wrong to be upset? What happened when you tried to speak up?

_____

_____

_____

When did you first learn to suppress anger to stay safe?

Was it in childhood? A relationship? A job? What did you trade in order to stay accepted?

_____

_____

_____

What are you *still* angry about that you haven't given yourself permission to feel?

List it without censoring. This is not about judgment. It's about truth.

_____

_____

_____

What does your anger want you to notice?

What boundary was crossed? What lie was told? What part of you was denied?

_____

_____

_____

Have you confused anger with bitterness, rebellion, or failure?

What if your anger is actually your *wisest emotion*—the one asking for justice, not revenge?

_____

_____

_____

What would it look like to let your anger speak—not to destroy, but to *reveal*?

What would it say if it were safe? Who would it confront? What would it demand?

_____

_____

_____

Now Step Back and Look

Anger is clarity in a world that told you to shut your mouth and smile. It is the part of you that knows this wasn't okay—and refuses to let it slide. Your abusers may want you to stay quiet. Your workplace may want you to stay small. Your family may want you to keep the peace.

But peace that comes at the cost of truth isn't peace—it's bondage. Let your anger tell you what was violated. Let it remind you of what you deserved and didn't receive. Let it burn—not to destroy you, but to refine you.

This isn't about staying angry forever. It's about finally telling the truth without flinching. Because when you stop denying your pain, you start reclaiming your power. You're not broken for being angry—you're finally waking up.

> In my own writing, I wrote through my anger. In releasing each heart-hurt—whether from myself or imposed on me—I felt freer. I wrote despite self-ridicule, judgment, and condemnation. All of the hurt poured out onto the pages: all of the anger, all of the shame.
>
> I had never written a book before. I didn't know what the heck I was doing. My spirit told me I had a strong story, but my writing? It was that of a child—an impetuous child who still needed to be right, still needed to be affirmed, still needed to be valued.

I struggled for months, trying to edit my book by myself, feeling defeated each day as I looked at my computer with all the red-marked errors spread through the chapters. It felt overwhelming. An accomplishment so close, yet it seemed so far away.

And then, I did something I normally don't do—I asked for help. Help came in the form of a woman I met on a book-writing retreat. Her own path was very accomplished: an author, a filmmaker, and a former Purdue English professor.

I started working with Marya, and the fog lifted. She saw my story. She heard my words. She believed in my mission field. She believed that this book would resonate with many. That is when my anger started to wane. The stronghold that had gripped me deep in the pit of my soul began to loosen.

This is where denial began to break—the denial that what I had to say was important. As I found clarity, my passion returned. Her support was exactly what I needed to move through a very trying season in my life when I felt frozen.

You can feel your anger. You can express your anger. But don't expect to heal through it. It's only a tool. Healing takes peace. It takes humility. It takes honesty. And it takes diligence.

26

TIRED OF BEING TIRED

THE MIRROR WAS NEVER THE ENEMY

This is your call to truth. Not survival. Not performance. But peace.

You've walked through the wreckage. You've named the labels, the roles, the silences, the screams. You've looked shame in the face. You've stopped protecting people who never protected you. You've felt the weight of what was never yours to carry—yet you carried it anyway. Now it's time to stop scattering your truth across a thousand rooms. Now it's time to pull the mirror back and see the whole damn thing— not the curated image, not the version they liked, not the one who performed strength to avoid rejection. The full you: the girl they silenced, the man who raged, the child who was never protected, the adult who still shows up anyway. The addict. The forgiver. The fighter. The one who ran. The one who stayed. The one who lived. All of it belongs. All of it is you. And none of it disqualifies you from peace.

This is your call to action: put it all on one page. The names. The lies. The stories. The truths. Everything they called you. Everything you believed. Everything you now know was never yours to carry. Write it. Face it. Own it. Then stop obeying it. Because healing doesn't come from hiding. Healing comes when you stop begging for permission to be whole. It comes when you stop calling survival strength. It comes when you stop lying to yourself—even if no one else is watching.

So yes, this is for you. But it's also for them, for the ones who will finish this and still say, "I'm fine," "It wasn't that bad," "I'm just tired," "It's too late for me." No, it's not. If you're still lying to yourself after everything you've just seen—you're not broken. You're scared. You're stuck. But you are capable of more. You can still grow. You can still choose truth over comfort. You can still say, "I want to heal," even just a little. Even if all you can do today is admit that you're tired of carrying the lies that complex trauma has ruled your life without your permission.

Here's what healing actually looks like: it's not clean. It's not pretty. It's not for show. It's truth over image. Peace over performance. Self-acceptance over self-erasure. It's waking up and deciding you get to be you—unapologetically. Permanently. Fully. You—without the shame, the mask, or the need to explain. You don't owe anyone a sanitized version of your pain. You don't need another performance of progress. You need truth. You need peace. You need yourself. This is the takeback. This is the mirror turned outward and shattered, so you can finally turn inward and whole.

> You've done the work. And you're not done—because growth doesn't stop. Healing doesn't arrive once. It returns every time you choose truth instead of silence, every time you speak without apology, every time you show up in your life as you. So take the page. Write the names. Tell the truth. Reclaim your reflection. And walk in peace—not perfection, not performance—just you. And that's more than enough.
>
> Your mirror was never the enemy. It was just terrified of the freedom you might expose once you looked, explored, and then turned your back on it. So go. Walk in peace. Not performance. Not perfection. Just you. I can guarantee that's more than enough. You are more than enough. And that's a good thing. Be free. Know you are free. Say the truth. Live in the truth of your circumstances. Because from here on out—the only way is up. Awareness is not a cage you were placed in; it's a beginning of a new life.

27

THE TABLE IS SET

RECOVERY, BREAKING CHAINS, AND SAYING HELLO TO A NEW LIFE

*T*he table is set. It is no longer the table where silence ruled, where shame sat at the head, and where fear kept watch over every word. This table is different. It is not built on secrets. It is not held together by denial. It does not require you to pretend. This table is set in truth.

For years, the confessions stayed buried. The memories felt like poison. The shame spoke louder than love. But shame does not get the last word, and silence does not own the final chapter. What once chained you to the past now becomes the very proof of your survival. The breaking of those chains is not a theory. It is the sound of your voice finally being heard, the weight of your boundaries holding strong, the light of your restored mind shining where darkness used to dwell.

At this table, the stories you were told to hide are spoken aloud. The names that carried power over you lose their sting. The secrets lose their grip when they are confessed in the open. The restored memories that once crushed you now carry the evidence of healing. You no longer carry them alone.

Recovery is not a straight line. It is a rhythm—falling down and rising again, breaking and mending, surrendering and standing. But it is recovery all the same. What mattered most was not perfection but persistence. You said "no more" to what tried to break you, and "yes" to the One who never left you.

This is where the old chains fall. The chain of silence. The chain of image. The chain of abuse. The chain of guilt. The chain of shame. They do not bind you anymore.

And now, the table is set for something new. The chairs are pulled close, not for pretense, but for presence. There is room for honesty, for laughter, for tears, for faith, for joy. There is space to breathe without apology. The table is set for peace. The table is set for freedom. The table is set for the life you were always meant to live.

So say hello. Hello to a new mind. Hello to a new way of living. Hello to a voice no longer silenced. Hello to boundaries that hold. Hello to freedom that does not leave because you now possess the strength to name it and move past from shame.

The table is set. And you belong here.

This is the day I put my story in ink and claim it as mine.

I _____Confirm I completed this workbook and offer my personal Signature of Truth: No More Silence, No More Shame. I will start to heal. I will reach out to professionals that can help me heal. I will invest in myself. I am worth it.

Date: _____

There you have it, my first workbook. Yes- it is brutal. Yes- it's been alarming and highly uncomfortable at times. Yes – you pushed back , - maybe more than a few times. Trust me I did it right alongside of you – every step of the way. Every self-discovery I have overcome came from personal lived experience. I was actively "surviving" so well that I believed I was thriving. Toxic culture was draped in systemic dysfunction I had normalized to survive. I had been living in utter chaos in my mind, keeping it all together with plates spinning over my head. On one foot.

I was like an elaborate Paper Marche ball. Layers and layers of damage had to come off the top to even get to the heart of understanding myself and my emotions, reactions and anger at the injustice of the abuse that was imposed on me.

Every "ah-ha" moment came with tears, prayers and therapy. It's been exciting, exhilarating, scary, messy and a time of true reflection and discernment. It takes work to uncover hidden secret self-abusive patterns that survival has taught you brings esteem, safety and acceptance.

Embracing my diagnosis of Complex PTSD has cleared my eyes and allowed me to heal—not just heal a little, not just heal where others can see, but truly heal with a deeper understanding of how to live a better life. I boldly confirm that, second only to accepting Christ at age forty-nine, acknowledging and understanding my mental illness has saved and transformed my life.

And if you are so inclined, say hello to Christ, who sits at the head of my table—not shame, not silence, not fear. Only clarity. Only love.

Be well, - Jo

ABOUT THE AUTHOR

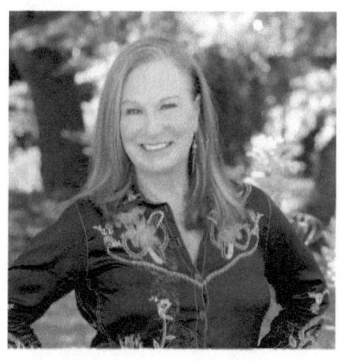 Joanne Richardson is the author of Virtue of Honor: Acquiring Truth—a memoir that gives childhood trauma a voice and testifies to resilience, redemption, and truth. Drawing from her own lived experiences, Joanne brings raw honesty to the page, breaking the silence around abuse, complex PTSD, and the long journey of healing.

Beyond writing, Joanne leads workshops and speaks publicly on mental health awareness, trauma recovery, and integrity in the workplace, equipping audiences with both education and encouragement.

Her faith in Jesus Christ is the foundation of her story. Every page, workshop, and talk reflects her conviction that true healing and freedom come through Christ alone.

Through her book, workshops, and speaking engagements, Joanne continues to empower others to confront painful truths, embrace their own stories, and find freedom on the other side of trauma.

www.ingramcontent.com/pod-product-compliance
Lightning Source LLC
Chambersburg PA
CBHW021039130626
46552CB00005B/1927